Bates

THE

POCKET GUIDE

TO THE

DSM-5™

DIAGNOSTIC

EXAM

THE
POCKET GUIDE
TO THE
DSM-5™
DIAGNOSTIC
EXAM

Abraham M. Nussbaum, M.D.

Director, Denver Health Adult Inpatient Psychiatry;
Assistant Professor, Department of Psychiatry,
University of Colorado School of Medicine

Washington, DC
London, England

Note: The authors have worked to ensure that all information in this book is accurate at the time of publication and consistent with general psychiatric and medical standards, and that information concerning drug dosages, schedules, and routes of administration is accurate at the time of publication and consistent with standards set by the U.S. Food and Drug Administration and the general medical community. As medical research and practice continue to advance, however, therapeutic standards may change. Moreover, specific situations may require a specific therapeutic response not included in this book. For these reasons and because human and mechanical errors sometimes occur, we recommend that readers follow the advice of physicians directly involved in their care or the care of a member of their family.

Books published by American Psychiatric Publishing (APP) represent the findings, conclusions, and views of the individual authors and do not necessarily represent the policies and opinions of APP or the American Psychiatric Association.

Manufactured in the United States of America on acid-free paper
17 16 15 14 13   5 4 · 3 2
First Edition

American Psychiatric Publishing
A Division of American Psychiatric Association
1000 Wilson Boulevard
Arlington, VA 22209-3901
www.appi.org

Library of Congress Cataloging-in-Publication Data
Nussbaum, Abraham M., 1975–
    The pocket guide to the DSM-5 diagnostic exam / Abraham M. Nussbaum. — 1st ed.
        p. ; cm.
    Pocket guide to the Diagnostic and statistical manual of mental disorders-5 diagnostic exam
    Pocket guide to the Diagnostic and statistical manual of mental disorders-five diagnostic exam
    Includes bibliographical references and index.
    ISBN 978-1-58562-466-9 (pbk. : alk. paper)
    I. American Psychiatric Association. II. Title. III. Title: Pocket guide to the Diagnostic and statistical manual of mental disorders–5 diagnostic exam. IV. Title: Pocket guide to the Diagnostic and statistical manual of mental disorders-five diagnostic exam.
    [DNLM: 1. Diagnostic and statistical manual of mental disorders. 5th ed. 2. Interview, Psychological—methods. 3. Mental Disorders—diagnosis. 4. Physician-Patient Relations. WM 141]
    RC470
    616.89'075—dc23   2013006020

British Library Cataloguing in Publication Data
A CIP record is available from the British Library.

Contents

Preface

The *Diagnostic and Statistical Manual of Mental Disorders* (DSM-5; American Psychiatric Association 2013) is an expansive manual of mental illness. For each illness, it provides diagnostic criteria and discusses the disorder from perspectives as diverse as development, genetics, and temperament. My book, *The Pocket Guide to the DSM-5 Diagnostic Exam,* is intended to serve as a map, as a pragmatic companion, for using DSM-5 in diagnostic interviews. Although this book is no replacement for either DSM-5 itself or psychiatric interview textbooks (see, e.g., MacKinnon et al. 2006; Shea 1998; Sullivan 1954), it describes a way to efficiently and effectively employ the DSM-5 criteria as part of a comprehensive diagnostic interview.

I interview patients daily with students, trainees, and fellow practitioners, and I wrote the book for interviewers at all levels of experience. The book follows the structure of DSM-5. So, in the first section, I introduce the diagnostic interview. The first and second chapters address the goals of a diagnostic interview. The third chapter provides an efficient structure for learning the diagnostic interview. The fourth and fifth chapters describe how DSM-5 alters the diagnostic interview. In the second section, I operationalized the DSM-5 diagnostic criteria for clinical practice. In the third section, I have included diagnostic tools and additional information.

Taken as a whole, this book helps you accurately diagnose a person in mental distress while establishing a therapeutic alliance, which remains the goal of any psychiatric encounter, even one as brief as a diagnostic interview.

Before beginning, I wish to acknowledge that a robust debate exists about whether or not the object of medical care is best construed as an ill patient under the care of a health professional or as an autonomous consumer of that professional's services (Emanuel and Emanuel 1992). Although this debate is fundamental, it is also outside the scope of the present book. In this book, because personhood precedes illness or consumption, I use the term *person* to describe the object of the initial diagnostic interview. When possible, I use gender-neutral terms for the person and the interviewer, but when doing so is grammatically awkward, I alternate between the universal feminine in one chapter and the universal masculine in the next chapter. When speaking about a person who has entered psychiatric treatment after an initial interview, I use the term *patient* because it acknowledges both the vulnerability of the person in treatment and the responsibilities assumed by mental health professionals when they care for patients (Radden and Sadler 2010). I use this term not to endorse medical paternalism but to emphasize that the particular and protected relationships that develop in clinical encounters are better described as therapeutic relationships than as therapeutic contracts.

Acknowledgments

This book began out of my fumbling attempts to speak with people in mental distress, and is designed to continue (and improve) those conversations, so I thank all the patients, students, and teachers I learned from along the way. Discretion prevents me from naming the patients. The passage of time impedes me from naming all the students. So I thank the teachers whose habits I try to emulate: Lossie Ortiz, Betsy Bolton, Andrew Ciferni, Stanley Hauerwas, Don Spencer, Sue Estroff, Amy Ursano, Gary Gala, David Moore, Julia Knerr, Karon Dawkins, Joel Yager, Eva Aagaard, and Robert House. Finally, I thank Melissa Musick and Melanie Rylander for reading (and improving) drafts of this book.

The author has no competing interests or conflicts to declare.

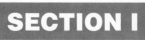

SECTION I

Chapter 1

Introduction to the Diagnostic Interview

When a person is experiencing mental distress, her first psychiatric encounter is often confusing or frightening. To a greater degree than in other areas of medicine, a person often has to overcome a series of obstacles before she is evaluated for mental distress (Radden and Sadler 2010). The obstacles can include access, expense, fear, and stigma, but once a person overcomes these particular hurdles, she deserves an encounter that establishes the nature of her suffering and initiates a working relationship. Although there are various ways to account for mental suffering, this book describes use of the fifth edition of the *Diagnostic and Statistical Manual of Mental Disorders* (DSM-5; American Psychiatric Association 2013), the newest version of the common language spoken by mental health professionals. DSM-5 has many perceptive critics (see, e.g., Phillips et al. 2012a, 2012b, 2012c), and I do not presume in this book that DSM-5 is flawless, but I do presume that DSM-5 offers a common way of organizing a psychiatric encounter into a diagnosis that contemporary professionals can understand (Kinghorn 2011).

Because the findings of a psychiatric examination are neither as obvious nor as well understood as, for example, a subluxated shoulder, mental health professionals need a common language like DSM-5 to describe these findings. Psychiatric findings are usually divided into *symptoms,* a person's subjective report of an abnormality, and *signs,* objective findings of an abnormality. These distinctions between signs and symptoms emphasize the source of a psychiatric finding, but the most important thing is not the provenance of a finding but how you use clinical judgment to weigh any signs and symptoms in your diagnosis (King 1982). Although signs are generally considered more telling than symptoms, because they are observed, both signs and symptoms are open to interpretation. When you observe a person crying, her tears may indicate grief or joy or grit trapped under a contact lens. A sign like tears has little meaning independent of the person who is crying.

Although many psychiatric signs and symptoms are particular to a specific mental illness, most are nonspecific—everyone has experienced sleepless nights and trouble concentrating—and most people experiencing a psychiatric sign or symptom do not have a mental illness. By their nature, psychiatric signs and symptoms often exist in the borderlands between what is normal and what is pathological (Pierre 2010). Clearly, interpreting these signs and symptoms is difficult, and the risk of misdiagnosis is real (Rosenhan 1973), so you have an ethical responsibility to diagnose the suffering person before you as accurately as possible (American Psychiatric Association 2010).

It is your responsibility to understand the relationship between the signs you observe, the symptoms you elicit, and their effect on the person you meet. The effects can be profound, because although all illnesses threaten bodily integrity (Cassell 1991), mental disorders can compromise a person's ability to think, feel, and act. Because these faculties are centrally connected with a person's agency, self, and identity (McHugh and Slaveny 1998), mental disorders are often experienced as a greater existential threat. So when you see a person for the first time, remember that she may be asking herself something like, "What is wrong with me? Am I going crazy?" When you listen well to a person's report and identify the nature of the suffering, you can provide the relief that comes from giving a name to nameless fears. You need to name suffering as accurately as you are able, and DSM-5 is a learned attempt to improve your clinical judgment as you characterize mental distress through the diagnoses of mental disorders.

DSM-5 improves the accuracy of psychiatric diagnoses by measuring the severity of a disorder, aligning diagnoses with the *International Classification of Diseases* (ICD) system, and incorporating recent advances in neurosciences (Kupfer and Regier 2010). DSM-5 was conceived by leaders of the American Psychiatric Association and other mental health groups a decade ago, but was ultimately crafted by many people organized into 6 study groups, 13 diagnostic work groups, and a task force of advocates, clinicians, and researchers (Regier et al. 2009). The resulting criteria were thrice made available online for public comment and field-tested for their reliability and validity (American Psychiatric Association 2013).

In addition to this public process, the signal advance of DSM-5 is the introduction of "dimensions," psychiatric symptoms that occur within and across specific disorders. Dimensions are discussed at length in Chapter 4, "Adventures in Dimensions," but in brief, they were introduced to reduce comorbidity and to begin moving toward a diagnostic system based on signs that indicate the dysfunction of neural circuits, rather than a diagnostic system based on symptoms. This marks a departure from previous DSM versions.

The authors of DSM began constructing diagnoses around the presence or absence of symptoms in the third edition (American Psychiatric Association 1980). This diagnostic model is sometimes called a *categorical model*, because a person either does or does not have a mental illness that fits into a diagnostic category, based on her symptoms. Since DSM-III, the diagnostic criteria have included little mention of the cause of a mental disorder, the so-called atheoretic principle, even when a cause was closely associated with a disorder (Wilson 1993). Focusing on the description rather than the cause of a disorder allowed mental health professionals who disagreed about the etiology of mental distress to work together. DSM-III proved very useful for mental health practice and research, so subsequent revisions maintained the categorical model. Its problems became more apparent over time, however, and DSM began to look like a birding guide, in which external characteristics identified the species to which a bird belonged, irrespective of the cause of these characteristics (McHugh 2007).

Richard Bentall, a British psychologist, once observed that because happy people are statistically rare, exhibit cognitive distortions like optimism, and experience a discrete cluster of symptoms, happiness is a mental disorder. Accordingly, Bentall proposed that people experiencing happiness be diagnosed with major affective disorder, pleasant type (Bentall 1992). Bentall was joking about the diagnosis but serious about his critique of a diagnostic system that was sometimes unable to distinguish the normal, but rare, from the pathological (Aragona 2009).

To respond to such concerns, the authors of DSM-5 added dimensional assessments, which will be new for most interviewers, while refining the categorical model that most current interviewers know. Because DSM-5 will be widely adopted, I wrote this book to guide both novice and seasoned interviewers as they conduct a DSM-5 diagnostic examination using both categorical and dimensional assessments. The book includes a practical discussion about initiating and developing a therapeutic alliance during a diagnostic examination (Chapter 2), spends several chapters observing how DSM-5 affects the diagnostic examination (Chapters 3–5), and continues with an operationalized version of DSM-5 for the purposes of conducting a diagnostic examination (Chapter 6). As we begin, it is useful to ask, "What is the goal of a diagnostic interview?"

Disorders Instead of *Illnesses* or *Disease*

When you conduct a diagnostic interview, you generate a diagnosis. The diagnoses generated by a DSM-5 interview are called *disorders,* rather than *diseases* or *illnesses.* All three terms describe impairments of normal functioning, but the DSM system uses *disorders* to acknowledge the complex interplay of biological, social, cultural, and psychological factors involved in mental distress.

Physicians usually think in terms of diseases, which can be described as pathological abnormalities in the structure and function of body organs and systems. Patients usually present with illnesses, their experience of pathological abnormalities or of being sick. From a distance, diseases and illnesses may seem like the same experience viewed from the different perspectives of patient and physician. However, consider a condition such as hypertension, which is often identified incidentally, without any associated clinical findings. To the diagnosing physician, hypertension is a chronic disease of the vasculature that increases the risk of stroke and a heart attack, but patients often do not recognize themselves as being sick or as having an illness. Conversely, a patient may present as feeling quite ill and describe herself as homesick, but physicians do not recognize this as a disease. Diseases and illnesses are often divergent experiences, rather than merely different perspectives, as anthropologists have repeatedly documented (Estroff and Henderson 2005).

An anthropologist can also tell you that these experiences are culturally constructed: different conditions will be recognized as diseases or illnesses in different places and times. However, to be recognized as suffering from a disease or an illness, an individual requires some kind of diagnosis, often a diagnosis from a physician.

When a particular culture recognizes a person as suffering from a condition that alters one's place in the community, the person enters what sociologist Talcott Parsons (1951) famously called the "sick role." Parsons observed that a person recognized as sick is exempted from normal social roles. Sick people do not have to perform their usual roles, but the degree of exemption from their social roles is relative to the nature and severity of their illness, as well as to their ages and cultural roles. To use contemporary examples, the child gets to stay home from school for mild fever and diarrhea, but the adult with back pain will receive disability only after experiencing years of refractory pain.

As part of the sick role, the sick person is usually not held responsible for her illness because sickness is believed to be beyond human control. Illness requires assistance to effect a change. So when a physician diagnoses a person with a sickness, the physician legitimizes her illness and admits her to the sick role (Parsons 1951). Admitting a person to a particular culture's sick role is part of what occurs when you diagnose a person's distress as a specific condition, and you need to remember that any diagnosis you assign to a person's distress has this cultural function.

Although all diagnoses have a cultural function, psychiatric diagnoses are especially complicated. Mental disorders result from biological, genetic, environmental, social, and psychological events, and these etiological factors are involved to varying degrees in different psychiatric diagnoses (Kendler 2012). Furthermore, because psychiatric diagnoses describe dysfunction in faculties believed to define one's personhood, they often constitute a threat to a person's sense of identity (Rüsch et al. 2005).

To recognize this complexity, the authors of DSM chose the term *disorder* to describe psychiatric diagnoses. *Disorder* can broadly be defined as a disturbance in physical or psychological functioning. The term is used elsewhere in medicine to describe genetic disorders and metabolic disorders. However, most diagnoses in medicine are called diseases rather than disorders, and naming psychiatric diagnoses as disorders reinforces a distinction between mental problems, *disorders,* and physical problems, *diseases* (Wallace 1994). We can see this when we consider that while a psychiatrist diagnoses a person with a "mental disorder," an internist does not diagnose a person with a "physical disease." Instead, an internist tersely diagnoses a person with a "disease," which illustrates how our use of the adjective "mental" before "disorder" implicitly endorses a division between the body and the mind.

The authors of DSM-5 addressed this concern by removing the multiaxial system, as we discuss in Chapter 5, "Key Changes in DSM-5." This takes away the difficulty, found in previous DSM versions, of documenting something like dementia on two separate portions of a person's diagnostic formulation (Wiggins and Schwartz 1994). Although this change removes one redundancy that reinforced divisions between the mind and body, the definition and limits of a disorder remain broad. They range from illicit behavior to a particular pathological process with a well-characterized etiology, genetics, and prevalence. Therefore, the ambiguity about what precisely a disorder *is* remains.

Still, all diagnoses are an abstraction of a person's experiences and bear the marks of the era in which they were constructed and employed. (To return to my previous example, hypertension was not diagnosed in the sixteenth century.) In this sense, using *disorder* to describe mental distress draws attention to how mental distress impairs a person's function, suggests the complex interplay of events that result in mental distress, and implicitly acknowledges the limits of our knowledge about the causes of mental distress. We simply do not know enough to be more precise. Instead, we can consider the ongoing use of *disorder* in our diagnostic systems as an opportunity for humility and a spur to further study.

The DSM-5 Definition of a Mental Disorder

The people you meet who have mental distress cannot simply wait for the precision that they and you desire—they deserve the best possible answers you can offer in the present moment. Richard Shweder (2003), the cultural anthropologist, famously observed that anything observed is incomplete from a single point of view, incoherent when observed from all points of view at once, and empty if observed from no point of view at all. You have to take a particular point of view, but with the understanding that despite being necessary, the point of view you take is necessarily incomplete. It is far easier to criticize definitions of a mental disorder than it is to construct an accurate, precise, and useful definition.

According to the authors of DSM-5, a mental disorder is "a syndrome characterized by clinically significant disturbance in an individual's cognition, emotion regulation, or behavior that reflects a dysfunction in the psychological, biological, or developmental processes underlying mental functioning." They distinguish a mental disorder from "an expectable or culturally approved response to a common stressor or loss, such as the death of a loved one." The authors caution, "Socially deviant behavior (e.g., political, religious, or sexual) and conflicts that are primarily between the individual and society are not mental disorders unless the deviance or conflict results from a dysfunction in the individual." This definition of a mental disorder, along with the authors' insistence that a diagnosis "have clinical utility" and "help clinicians to determine prognosis, treatment plans, and potential treatment outcomes for their patients" (American Psychiatric Association 2013), has several important implications for the diagnostic interview (Stein et al. 2010).

First, the definition characterizes a mental disorder as causing a clinically significant disturbance in a number of possible domains. This means that when you interview persons with mental distress, you need to explore the extent to which their distress significantly impairs their cognition, emotions, and behaviors. However, the definition does not characterize what constitutes a "significant" impairment. Without such precision, you need to define *impairment* with your patient based on how she functioned before the onset of the signs and symptoms with which she is presenting for evaluation. You might do this by asking the person to recall a time before the most recent onset of her distress and to describe the differences between her function at that point and in the present. Ideally, you will also obtain collateral information from people who know the person in multiple situations to help assess her premorbid ability and function. You may also want to use the World Health Organization Disability Assessment Schedule 2.0 (WHODAS 2.0), the disability assessment tool endorsed by the authors of DSM-5 (World Health Organization 2010), which is discussed in Chapter 11, "Selected DSM-5 Assessment Measures." Several other validated disability assessments are available, but whichever you use, you need to define *dysfunction* and *impairment*, along with their degree, individually for each person you evaluate.

Second, because the definition identifies dysfunction as occurring because of underlying disturbances in "the psychological, biological, or developmental processes underlying mental functioning," you need to assess all of these processes. The DSM-5 criteria offer clear guidance on how to elicit and organize symptoms of psychological processes, but provide less guidance for assessing biological and developmental processes. Because it is your responsibility to consider a person in full, you will need, at the least, to seek an understanding of the person's medical history and developmental stage. We briefly discuss ways to assess these processes in Chapter 3, "The 30-Minute Diagnostic Interview," and Chapter 8, "A Stepwise Approach to Differential Diagnosis."

Third, the definition excludes dysfunction that is in some way expected. This can include responses to events such as the death of an intimate or the loss of employment—that is, events that induce mental distress in many people. The DSM-5 definition mentions "culturally approved" responses but does not define what constitutes either a culture or its approval, which further points to your need to assess the relationship between the symptoms you elicit in a diagnostic interview and their context in a person's life. Therefore, you might ask the person, or her family, friends, partners, and peers, if her response is consistent with the responses of her culture, because you need to explore the cultural context in which the person with mental distress presents.

Fourth, the definition simultaneously excludes dysfunction caused by a disagreement between a person and her broader culture. A person's thoughts and behaviors may clearly be in conflict with those of her intimates or with her culture. Conflict in and of itself is not evidence of a mental disorder. A person can disagree with the leaders of her country, disengage from her faith community, or dislike her siblings without having a mental disorder. For a diagnostic interview, establishing a person's cultural expectations and baseline behaviors is important, especially when you are interviewing a person whose age, gender, culture, experience, faith, language, or lifestyle is different from your own—in short, almost everyone you meet. You should ask a person what her distress means rather than make assumptions about its meaning.

Fifth, the definition includes an important caveat: a diagnosis must be clinically useful. This caveat helps further distinguish DSM-5 from a birding guide, because even if a person endorses all the symptoms of a particular disorder, if the disorder does not usefully inform that person's diagnosis, treatment, or prognosis, then the diagnosis is considered inappropriate. This requirement for clinical utility speaks to the pragmatic nature of DSM-5, which is a diagnostic system designed to enable accurate and reliable communication of psychiatric findings, rather than to diagnose disorders simply for the sake of doing so.

The Questions Produced by a Diagnostic Interview

In reviewing the definition of a DSM-5 mental disorder, it becomes clear that the authors of DSM-5 left much undefined. This lack of definition necessitates, as happens so often in psychiatry, the exercise of practical wisdom (Radden and Sadler 2010). In the diagnostic interview, it means applying diagnostic categories to the irreducibly particular person before you. To define a mental disorder for the person before you, you need to seek a thorough understanding of her as a person. While a good diagnostic interview produces a diagnosis, it also generates questions you will need to ask as you seek understanding. These questions can relate to diagnosis, treatment, and prognosis.

At the conclusion of any diagnostic interview, you should be able to generate a list of additional information you need for a more concrete diagnosis. This additional information can be as straightforward as collateral information from people who know your patient in other contexts, including reports from past psychiatrists, psychologists, therapists, counselors, primary care physicians, pastors, employers, coworkers, teachers, peers, friends, family, partners, and spouses. At times, you may wish to address particular areas of concern by administering additional diagnostic tests, such as physical or neurological examinations, or neuropsychological or personality tests. Before you administer additional tests, you should understand the strengths and limitations of each test and consider how a positive or a negative test result will change your therapeutic relationship. Finally, it is always useful to seek further understanding of a person's coping strategies and her understanding of the etiology and treatment of mental distress.

Although DSM-5 is not a treatment manual, the diagnostic interview is a time to consider whether and which treatment is indicated. In fact, with experience, you can begin treatment in the interview by incorporating some basic therapeutic techniques into your diagnostic interview. Many teachers recommend a classic text, *The Psychiatric Interview in Clinical Practice* (MacKinnon et al. 2006), to learn how to organize a psychiatric interview for the personality structure of your patient. If you do not yet feel able to introduce therapeutic techniques into your diagnostic interview, you should at least begin mentally formulating the case and identifying resources keyed to the person's particular problems and strengths as you interview her. Ways to do so are discussed in the next few chapters.

Finally, DSM-5 offers nothing in the way of prognosis, to help a patient know what to expect as sequelae of the treatment you recommend. You ought to offer reasonable hope to the person you interview. This hope should be informed by an evidence-based review of the scientific literature, your clinical wisdom, and your understanding of the person's premorbid functioning and of the resources available to her.

Conclusion

Critics of DSM-5 are concerned that it will be used as a psychiatric checklist rather than as a means for a comprehensive examination (McHugh and Slaveny 2012). DSM-5 certainly can be received and used that way. You can also employ it as one part of a diagnostic interview that both characterizes the distress a person describes and helps in beginning to understand the person who describes the distress. Despite its critics, nothing about DSM-5 itself precludes you from conducting a comprehensive examination. It is true that DSM continues to rely on the experiences and symptoms reported by a person, but you can receive this as an implicit acknowledgment of the limits of the available knowledge about mental distress. In this fashion, your use of DSM-5 reflects your orientation toward the well-being of your patients, as well as your humility and your willingness to revise your opinions as you gain further insight. In short, you can use a DSM-5 diagnosis both as an invitation to understand a person's mental distress and as the beginning of a conversation rather than its conclusion.

Chapter 2

Alliance Building During a Diagnostic Interview

Every encounter with a person, even the first meeting, should be therapeutic. How can you accomplish this goal, especially within the context of a diagnostic interview? As discussed in Chapter 1, "Introduction to the Diagnostic Interview," part of your response to a patient's suffering is to accurately diagnose his mental distress. Naming a person's distress is itself beneficial. Although your responsibilities may begin with an accurate diagnosis, they extend to establishing a relationship in which you and your patient are mutually committed to his well-being. This relationship, called a *therapeutic alliance*, can be initiated even in a diagnostic interview.

The heart of all psychiatric treatments is the therapeutic alliance. This alliance is established when a patient identifies treatment goals and you ally yourself with the patient in pursuit of those goals. That is, you form an alliance between yourself and your patient with the goal of mobilizing healing forces within your patient by psychological means. Your ability to form these alliances profoundly influences the efficacy of your work for the patient, as well as your satisfaction with this work (Summers and Barber 2003).

If you want to know why a therapeutic alliance is important, I recommend that you read Jerome and Julia Frank's *Persuasion and Healing: A Comparative Study of Psychotherapy* (Frank and Frank 1991), in which the authors consider why different forms of therapy—psychoanalysis, cognitive-behavioral therapy, group therapy, and Alcoholics Anonymous—as well as shamanistic encounters and religious faith can all effectively motivate change. The authors observe that most aspects of a person cannot be changed because most people have a fairly fixed set of assumptions about themselves and the world. If these assumptions are fixed, why do people seek out mental health practitioners? According to the Franks, people have maladaptive assumptions about themselves and the world that repeatedly fail. These repeated failures induce demoralization. The Franks write that the "major sources of demoralization are the pathogenic meanings patients attribute to feelings and events in their lives....Effective psychotherapies combat demoralization by persuading patients to transform these pathogenic meanings to ones that rekindle hope, enhance mastery, heighten self-esteem, and reintegrate patients with their groups" (Frank and Frank 1991, p. 52). Even during a diagnostic interview, you can identify maladaptive assumptions and the resulting demoralization. You can also rekindle hope.

How? The Franks observe that all effective forms of therapy identify a socially sanctioned healer, a demoralized sufferer who seeks relief from the healer, and a circumscribed relationship in which they meet. To provide therapy, you must identify with a particular theory and have an appropriate confidence in it.

Why? The Franks conclude that therapy is a kind of rhetoric in which you stimulate emotional arousal to transform the meaning of an event. That transformation can occur only if you can offer the patient a conceptual framework for making sense of his maladaptive assumptions and the resulting demoralization. You can effectively invoke serotonin receptors or the superego, so long as the framework is compelling to the patient and to you. You can begin this process in the initial interview (Alarcón and Frank 2011).

Think about your own life: Did you ever work with a teacher or coach who helped you master a skill you could not learn on your own? How were you motivated? What was your relationship with the motivator? Now think about a teacher or coach for whom you underperformed. What was the nature of that relationship?

Your own goal should be to foster relationships that help people make therapeutic changes in their lives, changes they could not make outside the relationship. A great example of someone forming an effective therapeutic alliance in a medical context is presented in the movie *Lars and the Real Girl* (Oliver 2007), in which Ryan Gosling plays a young man with a delusion. His physician, played by Patricia Clarkson, ably builds a relationship that allows her patient to gracefully give up his delusion.

This is not to say that you need to mimic Patricia Clarkson, or anyone else for that matter. During my residency training, many of us residents went through a painful period in which we began talking in faux therapist voices. We would greet each other guardedly, fearful that expressing any emotion or personal thought would somehow betray our insecurities and faults. The less confident residents bought tweed jackets and parroted our faculty. The more confident residents quickly moved beyond this stage and established their own styles. They showed me that a gregarious Texan, a laconic Ohioan, and a mannered South Carolinian could all be effective if they could connect with their patients.

If accurately applying the DSM-5 diagnostic criteria in all their specificity is the *science* of psychiatric interviewing, then the *art* is forming a therapeutic alliance. In an effective diagnostic interview, you conduct a form of rudimentary psychotherapy in which you instill hope and provide appropriate support to a demoralized patient. Your goal should be to initiate therapy as you assess a patient because this helps reinforce his intentionality (Mundt and Backenstrass 2005). The purpose of this chapter is to discuss efficient ways to form a therapeutic alliance during a DSM-5 diagnostic interview.

Practical Tips for Alliance Building in a Diagnostic Interview

In their analysis of how therapeutic encounters work, the Franks found that "effectiveness is primarily a quality of the therapist, not of a particular technique" (Frank and Frank 1991, p. 166). If you have an ideological commitment to a particular technique, their viewpoint may be discouraging, but it can also have a positive effect by encouraging you to take action to cultivate your skill as a therapist, because all therapies share the core skill of forming therapeutic alliances. As you become better able to form therapeutic alliances, you will improve your ability to practice any form of psychotherapy.

Your ability to form an alliance, however, will be shaped by a person's experiences before he even meets you. When you meet someone in the emergency department, he may have waited hours, even days, to see you, so the encounter may be terse and tense. When you meet a person in the office of his longtime family doctor, he may be trusting and tranquil. But these behaviors cannot be anticipated for all individuals. People bring to your encounter both conscious and unconscious associations about the place you meet and your role in that place. You cannot control those associations, but you can be aware of them. Before you meet a person for the first time, try to ascertain how he arrived at your meeting place, how long he waited to see you, and what he hopes to attain from your encounter.

As you approach a person for an interview, you can begin forming the alliance, before you even speak, by taking some practical steps. If you provide an environment in which people are safe enough to speak about intimate matters, you implicitly increase their trust in you. Ideally, the environment includes a comfortable chair for each of you, positioned so that you can make or avoid eye contact as necessary. This setup encourages conversation. Sitting with a patient has been shown to increase his perception of the time you spend with him (Johnson et al. 2008).

Because you never know how someone will respond to your presence, it is a good practice to sit closest to the exit in case you need to leave abruptly. Indeed, sometimes a person may be too agitated to tolerate sitting with you. Therefore, you should practice universal precautions for the diagnostic interview when meeting a person for the first time, to help ensure the safety of patient, practitioner, and staff. If staff members check a person into a room before you meet him, it can be helpful to ask the staff members about their sense of his behaviors and emotional state to ascertain if it is safe to conduct the interview alone. Although it is easier to preserve the confidentiality of a person's interview if you interview him alone, it is prudent to interview him with appropriate professional assistance if he is so upset that you fear for his safety or your own. If you will be accompanied during the interview, explain the purpose of your encounter to your companion before you meet the person or begin the interview.

Whether you approach the person with assistance or on your own, it helps to dress with care to signify your respect. Similarly, many interviewers have tissues or a glass of water available in case a person becomes tearful; providing small aids to a person in distress can be reassuring (Yager 1989).

Once you are ready to begin, you should initiate the conversation with a statement that advances the therapeutic alliance. An interviewer might simply say, "I am Dr. Chatterjee. I read your chart but would like to know more about you. What do you like to be called?" This brief statement communicates your name and your preparation for the meeting. It then invites the patient to identify himself as he chooses. An opening like this simultaneously indicates that you are prepared for your meeting but aware of the limits of your knowledge. Ideally, the patient will then present a coherent and comprehensive account of his current problem and its relationship to past experiences. Although this ideal rarely occurs, you should always listen to a person for 2–3 minutes as you begin a diagnostic interview, as I discuss in Chapter 3, "The 30-Minute Diagnostic Interview."

If you listen actively, you can further advance the therapeutic alliance, because active listening communicates respect for a patient and his concerns. As you listen, you should adopt a neutral but caring posture that communicates your attention and concern without committing to a particular interpretation of the patient's account. You are committed to the patient and his well-being, not to his interpretation of events. Therefore, you should avoid a premature rush to either judgment or solutions, both of which may seem like shortcuts to building an alliance but often commit you to an interpretation that is not borne out by further information.

Instead, you can build the alliance by using nonverbal cues, such as head nodding, facial expressions, appropriate eye contact, and other signs of active listening (Robertson 2005). Although expressing sympathy is appropriate, especially when a patient reports an event that causes him visible distress, you should never express sympathy with statements like, "I know what you are going through," because you want to maintain the focus on the patient you are interviewing. Instead, you can show empathy—which is both the cognitive act of recognizing someone in need and the affective act of sharing his suffering (Davies 2001)—through your facial expressions and by providing reassurance when appropriate. If the person expresses fear that he is "doing it wrong," reassure him briefly: "You are doing fine" (Morrison and Muñoz 2009). In a diagnostic interview, you want to manifest empathy and warmth toward your patient through active listening by cultivating a style that is at once courteous, conversational, and comprehensive.

Alliance Building Through Cultural and Social History

A therapeutic alliance is also established by asking questions. I discuss the questions specific to a DSM-5 interview in Chapter 3, "The 30-Minute Diagnostic Interview," and Chapter 6, "The DSM-5 Diagnostic Interview," but here it is important to consider questions that will provide a framework to understand the psychiatric signs and symptoms you will elicit. These framing questions simultaneously generate clinical information while building the therapeutic alliance. To build an alliance, you must express concern about a patient's well-being, not only about how he is adhering to treatment (Weiden 2007) or how well his symptoms and behaviors fit the criteria for a specific mental disorder. In a diagnostic interview, you can express concern about someone's well-being directly, by saying something like, "I hope you're okay," but it is especially helpful to express concern in a manner that simultaneously helps you better understand the patient. There are many ways to do so, but I review two here. In the first instance, you build the alliance by asking about the patient's cultural experience of illness. In the second instance, you build the alliance by asking for an abbreviated version of his social history. By either method, you engage him as a person before engaging him as a patient.

The psychiatrist and anthropologist Arthur Kleinman spent his career reflecting on what it means for people of different cultures to meet during times of illness. He found that physicians often assume they know the meaning an illness has for an ill person. When Kleinman and his colleagues asked about, rather than assumed, the meaning of an illness, they heard something quite distinct from what they expected. Based on these findings, Kleinman encourages physicians to act like anthropologists and ask a person what his illness means, using these 10 questions (adapted from Kleinman et al. 1978, p. 256):

1. What do you think caused your problem?
2. Why do you think it started when it did?
3. What do you think your sickness does to you?
4. How does it work?
5. How severe is your sickness?
6. Will it have a short or long course?
7. What kind of treatment do you think you should receive?
8. What are the most important results you hope to receive from this treatment?
9. What are the chief problems your sickness has caused for you?
10. What do you fear most about your sickness?

By asking these questions, you gain valuable insight into how someone understands his mental distress and his cultural account of illness. In addition, you also build the alliance, by exhibiting a sense of curiosity and humility about the patient before you and his particular culture. The authors of DSM-5 implicitly endorse this approach by including two tools for assessing culture, the Outline for Cultural Formulation and the Cultural Formulation Interview. (The latter is discussed further in Chapter 4, "Adventures in Dimensions," and Chapter 11, "Selected DSM-5 Assessment Measures.")

If this approach seems too involved, one of my teachers, Joel Yager, recommends asking four simple social history questions:

1. Where do you live?
2. With whom do you live?
3. How do you spend your days?
4. How do you support yourself?

These four simple questions allow you to simultaneously gather data for the social history and implicitly assess the patient's psychosocial functioning. These neutral, open-ended questions give you a sense of the patient's material, social, economic, and communal existence. They provide a context for the symptoms you elicit later and at the same time build an alliance by implicitly addressing him as a person before you address his status as a patient.

Alliance Building Through Role Relationships

As you listen to a patient, it is common to hear what he is saying and, with experience, how he is saying it. You should eventually ascertain to whom he is speaking. In any conversation, people unconsciously assume role relationships. In a clinical encounter, a patient may receive you as a loving parent, as a cruel peer, or as an indifferent partner. A skilled therapist quickly ascertains how a patient conceptualizes the people he trusts and distrusts. In a good therapeutic alliance, you modulate your interview in response to a patient's needs.

This is a complicated skill, and learning it requires practice beyond the scope of this book. The best model for this remains Otto Kernberg's (1984) classic text, *Severe Personality Disorders*. The entire book, especially the first two chapters, is important for anyone interested in considering how to understand role relationships during a diagnostic interview. Drawing on Kernberg's work, I recommend that as you interview a patient, you silently ask yourself these questions:

- Who is this patient addressing?
- How is this patient experiencing me?
- How is this patient portraying himself?
- How does this patient describe the personality of, and his relationship with, his mother, father, siblings, previous therapist, or other important caretaker?

Learning to reflect on how a patient perceives and relates to other people efficiently advances your understanding of him. This kind of reflection also deepens the therapeutic alliance. You can cultivate this habit—thinking about and with other people—even during a diagnostic interview.

Conclusion

An important goal is to use DSM-5 not as a checklist but as part of a thorough diagnostic interview. People do not seek your assistance to determine if their mental distress meets diagnostic criteria. The core of the diagnostic interview is not an assessment of the psychiatric symptoms, but rather the formation of a therapeutic alliance, which involves learning to think with your patient. I think of a therapeutic alliance as a relationship in which you and a patient in distress work together to reduce his distress and increase his sense of agency. In an effective diagnostic interview, you conduct a form of rudimentary psychotherapy in which you instill hope and provide support to a demoralized patient. There are many practical steps you can take to form a therapeutic alliance, including using the basic techniques of an anthropologist, a social historian, or a psychoanalyst.

Chapter 3

The 30-Minute Diagnostic Interview

If you are efficient and empathetic, you can elicit the essential psychiatric symptoms and personality traits of a person with mental distress or illness in 30 minutes. To do so, you will have to practice.

In the recent past, preparing for the oral examination required for board certification in psychiatry fostered this skill. At the end of her training, a psychiatry resident engaged in a series of mock board exams, in which she spent 30 minutes evaluating a person she had never met. A senior psychiatrist watched in wordless judgment. The process initially made the resident anxious and worried about what the senior psychiatrist was thinking, but after completing several exams, she became less anxious and more confident in her interview skills.

During mock board exams, a resident honed her interview skills so that she was well prepared when it was time for the oral boards. When she traveled to a distant city and interviewed a single stranger while two senior psychiatrists she had never met silently assessed her proficiency, she was ready. The oral boards helped a young psychiatrist break the bad habit of assuming full knowledge of a person based on the medical records the psychiatrist had read before the first meeting. The process improved interview skills by forcing the practitioner to efficiently engage a patient in the initial encounter.

Although the external oral boards have been replaced (see Chapter 10, "The American Board of Psychiatry and Neurology Clinical Skills Evaluation"), residents and other interviewers still need ways to learn an organized psychiatric examination. When I prepared for my own oral boards, I read a number of interview books (Carlat 2005; MacKinnon et al. 2006; Morrison and Muñoz 2009; Shea 1998; Sullivan 1954; Zimmerman 1994) and adapted the advice into a timed outline for a 30-minute diagnostic examination. I practiced this exam 30 times until it became second nature, and I used it to pass my board exams.

Since then, I have taught this version of the diagnostic examination to residents and students, modifying it along the way to account for DSM-5. The outline, provided in the next section of this chapter, is timed and includes both general guidance and italicized question prompts. As you use the outline, it is important to avoid becoming a psychiatric robot, spitting out a screening question at a preordained time regardless of the patient before you. For example, asking, "I hear you are suicidal, but can you spell *world* backwards?" demonstrates more attention to your need for information than to the specific person before you. Rather, you should tailor your examination to the patient presenting with distress. A more organized patient may offer a concise history that you only need to clarify, whereas a patient displaying signs of mania or psychosis may be so disorganized that you will have to structure the interview. To tailor the interview, you must first learn to construct it. While you are developing your own interview style, it helps to practice a formal version until it becomes a habit. I recommend practicing a timed version of this exam. The 30-minute diagnostic interview may seem forced at first, but gradually it provides the underlying infrastructure for a conversational interview.

Outline of the 30-Minute Diagnostic Interview

The interview outline below includes headings that indicate the time allotted for the following portion of the interview (boldface type), instructions to the interviewer (roman type), and statements that are questions for the interviewer to ask (italic type).

Minute 1

Introduce yourself to the person. Ask how she would like to be addressed. Set expectations for how long you will meet and what you will accomplish. Then ask, *Why are you in psychiatric treatment?*

Minutes 2–4

Listen. A person's uninterrupted speech displays much of her mental status, guides your history taking, and builds the alliance. Although you may be tempted to interrupt or begin asking questions, with experience you will find that allowing the person to talk initially without interruptions gives you more information about her than the answers to your questions will. Depending on the nature of the illness, some people will be unable to fill this time; their inability to do so also reveals valuable information regarding their mental status and distress. In cases where the person does not speak spontaneously, you may have to use prompts and proceed to the history of the present illness.

Minutes 5–12

History of present illness.   Your questions should follow the DSM-5 criteria, as operationalized in Chapter 6, "The DSM-5 Diagnostic Interview," and summarized in Chapter 7, "A Brief Version of DSM-5." Additionally, you should focus on what has changed recently—the "why now?" of the presentation. As you do, seek understanding of precipitating events: When did the patient's current distress begin? When was the last time she felt emotionally well? Can she identify any precipitating, perpetuating, or extenuating events? How have her thoughts and behaviors affected her psychosocial functioning? How does she view her current level of functioning, and how is it different from what it was days, weeks, or months ago?

Past psychiatric history.   *When did you first notice symptoms? When did you first seek treatment? Did you ever experience a full recovery? Have you ever been hospitalized? How many times? What was the reason for those hospitalizations, and how long were you hospitalized? Do you receive outpatient mental health treatment? Do you take medications for a mental illness? Which medicines have helped the most? Did you have any adverse side effects to any medications? What was the reason for stopping prior medications? How long were you taking each medication, and how often did you take it? Do you know the name, strength, and number of doses per day of medicines you're currently taking, including over-the-counter and herbal medicines? Have you ever received injectable medications or electroconvulsive therapy?*

Safety.   Students and residents may feel uncomfortable asking these questions and may worry that they will upset people or even give them ideas about ways to hurt themselves or others. These fears are largely unfounded, and with practice you will find these questions become much easier to ask. It is important to remember that one of the biggest predictors of future behavior is past behavior, so asking about prior episodes of violence to self and others is required for an overall risk assessment. *Do you frequently think about hurting yourself? Have you ever attempted to kill yourself? How many attempts have you made? What did you do? What medical or psychiatric treatment did you receive after these attempts? Do you often have times when you become so upset that you make or even act upon verbal or physical threats to hurt other people, animals, or property? Have you ever been aggressive to people or animals, destroyed property, deceived other people, or stolen things?*

Minutes 13–17

Review of systems. The psychiatric review of systems is a brief overview of common psychiatric symptoms that you may not have elicited in the history of present illness. If a person answers affirmatively to these questions, you should explore further using the DSM-5 criteria, as modeled in Chapter 6.

MOOD. *Have you been feeling sad, blue, down, depressed, or irritable? Have you lost interest in, or do you get less pleasure from, the things you used to enjoy? Have there been times, lasting at least a few days, when you felt the opposite of depressed, when you were very cheerful or happy and this felt different from your normal self?* (See "Depressive Disorders," pp. 77–81, or "Bipolar and Related Disorders," pp. 72–76, in Chapter 6.)

PSYCHOSIS. *Have you seen visions or other things that other people did not see? Have you heard noises, sounds, or voices that other people did not hear? Do you ever feel like people are following you or trying to hurt you in some way? Have you ever felt you had special powers, such as reading other people's minds? Have you ever been listening to the radio or TV and felt it was referring to you?* (See "Schizophrenia Spectrum and Other Psychotic Disorders," pp. 68–71, in Chapter 6.)

ANXIETY. *During the past several months, have you frequently been worried about a number of things in your life? Is it hard for you to control or stop your worrying? Are there specific objects, places, or social situations that make you feel very anxious or tearful? A panic attack is a sudden rush of intense fear that comes on from out of the blue for no apparent reason, or in situations where you did not expect it to occur. Have you experienced recurrent panic attacks?* (See "Anxiety Disorders," pp. 82–86, in Chapter 6.)

OBSESSIONS AND COMPULSIONS.   *Do you frequently experience unwanted images, thoughts, or urges? Are there any physical acts you feel like you have to do in order to avoid or reduce the distress associated with these unwanted images, thoughts, or urges?* (See "Obsessive-Compulsive and Related Disorders," pp. 87–89, in Chapter 6.)

TRAUMA.   *What is the worst thing that has ever happened to you? Have you ever experienced or witnessed an event in which you were seriously injured or your life was in danger, or you thought you were going to be seriously injured or endangered? I am going to ask you a very personal question and if you are not comfortable answering, please let me know: Have you ever been physically, emotionally, or sexually abused?* (See "Trauma- and Stressor-Related Disorders," pp. 90–94, in Chapter 6.)

DISSOCIATION.   *Everyone has trouble remembering things sometimes, but do you ever lose time, forget important details about yourself, or find evidence that you took part in events you cannot recall? Do you ever feel like people or places that are familiar to you are unreal, or that you are so detached from your body that it is like you are standing outside your body or watching yourself?* (See "Dissociative Disorders," pp. 95–97, in Chapter 6.)

SOMATIC CONCERNS.   *Do you worry about your physical health more than most people? Do you get sick more often than most people?* (See "Somatic Symptom and Related Disorders," pp. 98–100, in Chapter 6.)

EATING AND FEEDING.   *What do you think of your appearance? Do you ever restrict or avoid particular foods so much that it negatively affects your health or weight?* (See "Feeding and Eating Disorders," pp. 101–104, in Chapter 6.)

SLEEPING.   *Is your sleep often inadequate or of poor quality? Alternatively, do you often experience excessive sleepiness? Do you frequently experience an irrepressible need to sleep or experience sudden lapses into sleep? Have you, or has a sleeping partner, noticed any unusual behaviors while you sleep? Have you, or has a sleeping partner, noticed that you stop breathing or gasp for air while sleeping?* (See "Sleep-Wake Disorders," pp. 107–114, in Chapter 6.)

SUBSTANCES AND OTHER ADDICTIONS.   *How often do you drink alcohol? On the average day when you have at least one drink, how many drinks do you have? Have you had any problems as a result of drinking? When you stop drinking, do you go through withdrawal?* Repeat for illicit and prescription drugs; begin by asking: *Have you ever experimented with drugs?* After asking about drugs, ask:

Do you bet, wager, or gamble in a way that interferes with your life? (See "Substance-Related and Addictive Disorders," pp. 129–158, in Chapter 6.)

PERSONALITY.   *When anyone reflects on their life, they can identify patterns—characteristic thoughts, moods, and actions—that began when they were young and have since occurred in many personal and social situations. Thinking about your own life, can you identify patterns like that which have caused you significant problems with your friends or family, at work, or in another setting?* (See "Personality Disorders," pp. 165–175, in Chapter 6.)

ELIMINATION.   *Have you repeatedly passed urine or feces onto your clothing, your bed, the floor, or another inappropriate place?* (See "Elimination Disorders," pp. 105–106, in Chapter 6.)

Minutes 18–23

Past medical history.   *Do you have any chronic medical problems? Have these illnesses affected you emotionally? Have you ever undergone surgery? Have you ever experienced a seizure or hit your head so hard you lost consciousness? Do you take any medications for medical illness? Do you take any supplements, vitamins, or over-the-counter or herbal medicines regularly?*

Allergies.   *Are you allergic to any medications? Can you describe your allergy?*

Family history.   *Have any of your relatives ever had nervousness, a nervous breakdown, depression, mania, psychosis or schizophrenia, problems resulting from excessive drinking or drug abuse; made suicide attempts; or required psychiatric hospitalization?*

Developmental history.   *Do you know if your mother had any difficulties during her pregnancy or delivery? What were you like as a child? Did you have any problems during your early childhood? When did you reach puberty, and how did you feel about it?*

Social history.   *Did you have any behavioral or learning problems during your early childhood? When you started school, did you have trouble relating socially or keeping up academically with your classmates because of behavioral or learning problems? How far did you make it in school? Who lived in your home during your childhood? Was a religious faith part of your upbringing? Currently? How do you support yourself? How did you support yourself previously? What is the longest period of time you have stayed at one job? What jobs have you held in the last 5 years? Have you ever served in the military? How long and what rank did you achieve? What discharge* *did you receive? Have you ever been arrested? Jailed? Imprisoned? What do you like to do? How do you spend your time online? What do you like about yourself? What do your friends like about you? Do you have any confidants? Are you sexually active? Are there any particular urges, fantasies, or behaviors that repeatedly cause you to feel intensely aroused? Have you been less interested in sex than usual or experienced difficulties in sexual performance? Are you uncomfortable with your gender? Do you feel safe in your current relationship? Are you, or have you been, married? Do you have any children? Who is currently with the children?*

Minutes 24–28

Mental status examination (MSE).   You should have already observed or obtained most of the pertinent data. See Chapter 9, "The Mental Status Examination: A Psychiatric Glossary," for a more detailed version of the MSE, which includes the following components:

- Appearance
- Behavior
- Speech
- Mood
- Affect
- Thought process
- Thought content
- Cognition and intellectual resources
- Insight/judgment: *What problems do you have? Are you sick in any way? What are your future plans?*

Mini-Mental State Examination (MMSE).   *It is obvious that people dealing with stress sometimes have difficulty concentrating or remembering. Have you had any problems of that sort? Help me, and the two of us together will get a handle on the extent to which you might be having those types of difficulties.* The MMSE comprises the following items: name, date and time, place, immediate recall, attention (counting backward from 100 by 7s, spelling *world* backward), delayed recall, general information (president, governor, five large cities), abstractions, proverbs, naming, repetition, three-stage command, reading, copying, and writing.

Minutes 29–30

Ask any follow-up questions. Thank the patient for her time and, if appropriate, begin discussing diagnosis and treatment.

Consider asking the following: *Have the questions I asked addressed your major concerns and problems? Is there anything important I missed or anything that I really should know about to better understand what you are going through?*

Presenting the 30-Minute Diagnostic Interview

If it takes a habituated sense of organization to complete this examination in 30 minutes, while altering its order and pace for each patient, it is comparatively easier to present your findings. Unlike the diagnostic interview, where you often have to supply the organization, the presentation has an organization that you have learned (or were supposed to have learned) in other contexts. The reality, however, is that formal presentations rarely occur outside of teaching services.

So why should you learn how to present the interview now? First, if you are a trainee, you will have to present a patient formally in order to earn board certification, as discussed in Chapter 10. Second, when you formulate and present your account of a patient's mental distress, you clarify your own thoughts, and this clarity improves your treatment plans and makes your written documentation more compelling to patients and other practitioners. When you successfully present a patient, you succinctly convey how well you understand her and her particular deficits and strengths. You also demonstrate your ability to organize the findings of your interview. To advance both skills, it is helpful to briefly review the following information about presenting a diagnostic interview.

Before you begin, gather your thoughts. Ask yourself if you can identify a central narrative from your interview. This is generally possible because most patients will present their distress as a story if you allow them to do so (Little 2005). If you listen well, you will hear patterns in these stories; common narratives include distress following a dangerous experience, the progressive decline from a chronic illness, recurrence in the context of a stressful situation or an interruption in treatment, interpersonal troubles that are consistent with previous episodes in a patient's history, and the development of behavioral patterns that cause distress. One way to think of clinical medicine is as a kind of practical problem solving through pattern recognition (Hunter 2005). If a narrative flows naturally from a patient's interview, organize your presentation around the narrative, because it will help you remember your findings and will be more engaging to your audience. However, always include evidence that both supports and discredits the narrative.

When you speak, present the patient as a kind of story, introducing her by name, age, gender, and a chief complaint, preferably with an illustrative quote from the patient. Follow with the history of her present illness, organized according to DSM-5 criteria, including pertinent information from the psychiatric review of systems. The middle portion of the presentation is straightforward—the past psychiatric history, the past medical history, family history, developmental history, and social history—but should be naturally connected to the central narrative of your presentation. In the last portion of the presentation, you interpret the interview, describing the patient's mental status examination, along with your differential diagnosis, assessment, and plan. As discussed in Chapter 8, "A Stepwise Approach to Differential Diagnosis," the differential diagnosis should include consideration of a patient's personality structure with deficits and strengths, substance use, cognitive ability or deficits, and other medical diagnoses that can mimic, alter, or otherwise complicate her treatment. You should always acknowledge your need for collateral, cross-sectional observation and serial examinations, as well as the limits of the history you obtained. Be sure to include predisposing biological, social, and psychological factors; current psychosocial stressors; and characteristic defenses in your formulation.

Finally, be prepared to offer an integrated workup, treatment plan, and prognosis. One way to do so is by following an inverted pyramid, in which the most pressing concerns are addressed at the beginning.

First, discuss any steps necessary to obtain or maintain safety. These should include the place where treatment should occur, the legal status of the patient, and her observation level. In any presentation, safety precedes all other concerns.

Second, address how the patient's physical health affects her treatment. In different settings, you might recommend a complete or focused physical examination, laboratory or imaging studies, referrals or consultations with other professionals, or nutritional or other treatments. Focus on the conditions that influence the patient's mental health.

Third, address any indicated psychiatric treatment, including psychoeducation, testing, therapeutic interventions, and medications. To the best of your ability, discuss the patient's past response to any medication; the cost of proposed medications; the known contraindications and interactions, along with any abuse potential; dose and dose titration; adverse effects and how you would ameliorate them; goal blood levels; the schedule of administration; whether the medications are best for short- or long-term use; and the cultural and legal consequences of treatment. Likewise, for any psychotherapy you recommend, describe the therapeutic problem, the recommended type of psychotherapy, the availability and affordability of therapy, the goal of therapy, and the motivation of the patient.

Fourth, address the patient's social and cultural needs. Discuss her strengths, living situation, significant relationships, employment, and community supports; the possibility of rehabilitative services; and any dependents. If you are concerned about the safety of a dependent, you should address it during the initial section of your formulation on safety.

Finally, assess the patient's prognosis in relation to symptoms, treatment response, comorbid medical diagnoses, duration of illness, previous response to treatment, compliance with treatment, availability and affordability of treatment, available social supports, and highest level of functioning.

As you present your findings, be appropriately self-critical. Admit any gaps or errors you recognize in your interview. Acknowledge your need for collateral and cross-sectional observations. Explain any deductions you made. Although the DSM-5 system is relatively more focused on symptoms than on signs, you should integrate a patient's signs into her symptoms and note any disjunction between signs and symptoms. Yet, make an effort to be succinct. Present the entire case without interrupting yourself, but be prepared for the examiner to interrupt you. Your goal should be to simultaneously present the patient you interviewed and show your audience how you think about a person experiencing mental distress.

Conclusion

When you conduct the diagnostic interview, you should listen actively. No matter how distracted or upset the patient is, you should always try to give her a few minutes to speak her own mind. As she speaks, listen to the content and form of her statements. What is she saying? How is she saying it? What is she not saying? How do her statements match her appearance? Summarize and clarify her concern, then organize the exam as necessary, modulating the structure and language of the interview to fit the needs of the patient before you. Ask clear and succinct questions. If the patient is vague, seek precision. If she remains vague, explore why. Do not ask permission to change the subject, but use transition statements, such as "I think I understand about this, but how about that?" Developing a supply of stock questions is helpful, which is precisely why I advise using this structured interview until it becomes a habit. Then you can use these questions to develop a conversational style for an interview in which a patient tells her story, you form an alliance with her, you gain insight into her thought process, and you gather the clinical data you need to make an accurate diagnosis. When you do so, you reduce the patient's alienation by making the strange more familiar.

Chapter 4

Adventures in Dimensions

Have you ever met a patient with major depressive disorder who has experienced panic attacks? I meet them weekly, but in DSM-IV-TR (American Psychiatric Association 2000), panic attacks were not part of the diagnostic criteria for major depressive disorder, even though people with depression often seek clinical assistance for panic. Using DSM-IV (or DSM-IV-TR), then, you could either ignore their panic or diagnose an additional disorder.

Have you ever struggled to decide how impaired a patient is by his schizophrenia? Some people with schizophrenia are profoundly disabled, some are high-functioning, and most people with schizophrenia live somewhere in between. In DSM-IV, you could describe the longitudinal course of a person with schizophrenia, but the specifiers only allowed you to describe the presence or absence of symptoms. DSM-IV did not provide a good way to describe which symptoms were present and how severe those symptoms were.

Have you ever met an anxious adolescent but been unsure how to efficiently determine if his anxiety was pathological? Using DSM-IV, you could certainly assess whether or not a particular adolescent met the criteria, but there were no screening tools available for general medical practices, where most anxious teenagers enter care.

DSM-5 addresses all three of these problems by introducing "dimensions," which are used to measure psychiatric symptoms. These dimensions are used to measure symptoms in three ways in DSM-5.

First, dimensions provide a way to acknowledge psychiatric symptoms that are not part of the diagnostic criteria of a patient's primary mental disorder. For example, if you treat a patient with major depressive disorder who also experiences panic attacks, you can add panic attack as a specifier to the diagnosis.

Second, dimensions allow psychiatrists to measure the magnitude of a symptom. For example, DSM-5 includes Clinician-Rated Dimensions of Psychosis Symptom Severity, which consist of 8 domains rated on a 5-point scale for their severity, rather than just their presence or absence (see Chapter 11, "Selected DSM-5 Assessment Measures, pp. 211–214).

Third, dimensions provide a way to screen for mental disorders in general clinical populations. For example, before evaluating an adolescent, a pediatrician could ask the patient to complete the DSM-5 Self-Rated Level 1 Cross-Cutting Symptom Measure, which is available in DSM-5 (Section III), as well as online at www.psychiatry.org/dsm5, and is discussed briefly in Chapter 11, "Selected DSM-5 Assessment Measures." If the pediatrician went over the results with the adolescent and a generalized anxiety disorder was suspected, the pediatrician could refer the adolescent to a child and adolescent psychiatrist, who could ask the patient to complete an adolescent-specific assessment tool for anxiety disorders, called PROMIS Emotional Distress–Anxiety (available at www.psychiatry.org/dsm5), which assesses how frequently the patient experiences symptoms of anxiety. A child and adolescent psychiatrist could subsequently ask the patient to complete the PROMIS Emotional Distress–Anxiety assessment before each encounter so an interviewer could chart the patient's progress.

According to the architects of DSM-5, the introduction of dimensions is their most important advance (Regier 2007). Why? Insightful critics have previously noted that the DSM diagnostic system could not always distinguish normality from pathology and one mental disorder from another (Kendell and Jablensky 2003). The architects of DSM-5 addressed these concerns by incorporating dimensions into their diagnostic system.

Consider the examples from above.

In the instance of a panic-ridden patient with major depressive disorder, the use of dimensions allows you to identify his problem without adding an additional diagnosis. This distinguishes a patient with depression who is experiencing panic problems from a patient with both panic disorder and major depressive disorder.

In the instance of a patient with schizophrenia, the use of dimensions allows a clinician to assess the severity of the patient's disorder, thus better distinguishing normality from pathology, and charting his progress. In a strictly categorical system like DSM-IV, a clinician determines only whether or not a person has a mental disorder. By adding dimensions, a clinician can grade the severity of a disorder as well as the particular symptoms that are most concerning to the patient, rather than simply declaring a patient does or does not have a disorder.

In the instance of the anxious adolescent, the use of dimensions leads to screening tools that supplement the diagnostic armamentarium of primary care providers and mental health practitioners alike.

How does the use of dimensions affect the diagnostic exam? The first implication is that you must screen for a wide range of psychopathology, because you cannot measure what you do not assess. The second implication is that you can record the symptoms you elicit and measure their severity. However, you need to keep in mind that dimensions supplement but do not replace the categories established in earlier DSM versions, as will be evident in the remainder of this chapter, which discusses some of the ways dimensions are (and are not) used in DSM-5.

Severity Ratings

DSM-5 provides severity rating scales for many disorders. Most of these scales are specific to a particular disorder, and many include a narrative description to indicate that a particular disorder is mild, moderate, or severe. For some diagnoses, such as alcohol use disorder, severity depends on the number of criteria endorsed by a patient. In other instances, severity is measured by the degree to which a patient requires support, as in autism spectrum disorder. Where appropriate, the severity ratings refer to specific measurements external to the mental status examination. For example, you assess the severity of anorexia nervosa by describing a patient's body mass index. In short, the various severity scales are designed to help you go beyond diagnostic categories to focus on the particular patient you are evaluating.

Perhaps the most groundbreaking of these tools is the Level of Personality Functioning Scale. This tool is discussed in Chapter 5, "Key Changes in DSM-5," and in Chapter 12, "Dimensional Diagnosis of Personality Disorders," but here I want to observe that it allows you to assess a wide range of personality traits, so that you can distinguish between, for example, the antagonism expressed by a person with antisocial personality disorder and that expressed by someone with narcissistic personality disorder. Interestingly, it also effectively offers a definition of mental health within DSM for the first time, with Level 0 (little or no impairment) on both the Self and Interpersonal scales implicitly indicating mental health.

The Level of Personality Functioning Scale was part of a proposed reconceptualization of personality disorders. This reconceptualization, discussed in Chapter 5, would have allowed an interviewer to identify the personality traits of a patient with remarkable specificity. While the authors of DSM-5 ultimately tabled the proposal in favor of the familiar categorical criteria for personality disorders, they thought highly enough of the proposal that they have included it among DSM-5's "Emerging Measures and Models." As this title suggests, if you familiarize yourself with the model described in Chapter 12, you will appreciate how a fully dimensional diagnostic system works. For now, DSM-5 uses dimensions in a more circumspect fashion.

Screening Tools

Most people will first seek help for mental distress from someone they already know. Within medicine, this will usually be a physician, nurse, or other professional who has typically not received specialized mental health training. Indeed, most mental health care occurs in the offices of primary care providers.

To address the gap between the mental health training that these providers possess and the volume of mental health care they provide, DSM-5 provides dimensional screening tools for use in primary care or mental health settings. These brief, easy-to-read, paper-based tools can be completed before a clinical encounter by the patient or someone who knows him well. Each tool has a series of short questions about recent symptoms; for example, "Have you been feeling more irritated, grouchy, angry than usual?" These screening questions assess core symptoms for the major diagnoses. For each symptom statement, a patient will assess how much this bothered him using a five-point scale: none (1), slight (2), mild (3), moderate (4), or severe (5). Each tool is designed to be easily scored. If a patient reports a clinically significant problem in any domain, you should consider a more detailed assessment tool available from www.psychiatry.org/dsm5.

As this example suggests, DSM-5 includes a hierarchy of screening tools and dimensional assessments. The initial assessment, the Level 1 Cross-Cutting Symptom Measure, is the screening tool described in the previous paragraph, and it is completed by the person seeking assessment, before an initial evaluation, or by the parent or guardian of a child. The adult version includes 23 questions assessing 13 domains of psychiatric symptoms. The child version includes 25 questions assessing 12 domains. For most, but not all, of the symptom domains screened for in the Level 1 Cross-Cutting Symptom Measure, there are separate Level 2 Cross-Cutting Symptom Measures for specific areas of concern like anxiety. When Level 1 and 2 assessments are used, they help an interviewer identify and address the presenting problems.

Once a person enters treatment as a patient, how do you measure his response and progress toward recovery? DSM-5 asks you to use these Level 2 Cross-Cutting Symptom Measures at your first evaluation of a patient in part so you can establish his baseline, and asks you then to revisit that assessment periodically to assess his progress. These measures assess dimensions (rather than diagnoses) that cut across diagnostic categories. These assessments will allow you, for example, to keep track of the depressive symptoms of a patient with schizophrenia in addition to his psychotic symptoms. Systematic use of these cross-cutting assessments will alert you to significant changes in a patient's symptomatology, will provide measurable outcomes for treatment plans, and, in aggregate, may alert researchers to lacunae in the current diagnostic system.

Cultural Assessments

DSM-5 similarly renews attention to the cultural specificity of mental distress. As I discuss in Chapter 1, "Introduction to the Diagnostic Interview," distress, disease, and illness are all profoundly shaped by cultural forces. As recommended in Chapter 2, "Alliance Building During a Diagnostic Interview," asking about a patient's cultural understanding of sickness and health is an efficient way to build a therapeutic alliance while gathering pertinent information. In addition, performing a cultural assessment also personalizes the diagnosis, which increases its accuracy (Bäärnhielm and Rosso 2009). In Section III of DSM-5, in "Cultural Formulation," the authors discuss cultural syndromes, cultural idioms of distress, and cultural explanations of perceived causes.

To use this cultural information in a diagnostic interview, it is beneficial to first define these terms. A *cultural syndrome* is a group of clustered psychiatric symptoms specific to a particular culture or community. The syndrome may, or may not, be recognized as an illness by members of a community or by observers. A classic example is *ataque de nervios,* a syndrome of mental distress characterized by the sudden onset of intense fear, often experienced physically as a sensation of heat rising in the chest, that may result in aggressive or suicidal behavior (Lewis-Fernández et al. 2010). The syndrome is often associated with familial distress in Latino communities (Lizardi et al. 2009). A cultural idiom of distress such as *ataque de nervios* is a way of discussing mental distress or suffering shared by members of a particular community. Finally, a cultural explanation of perceived cause provides an explanatory model of why mental distress or illness occurs (American Psychiatric Association 2013).

The Cultural Formulation Interview (CFI) is a structured tool, updated for DSM-5, to assess the influence of culture in a particular patient's experience of distress. The CFI can be used at any time during a diagnostic interview, but the DSM-5 authors suggest using it when a patient is disengaged during an interview, when you are struggling to reach a diagnosis, or when you are laboring to assess the dimensional severity of a diagnosis (American Psychiatric Association 2013). Although use of the CFI has been mostly studied in immigrant communities (Martínez 2009), you should not limit its use to situations in which you perceive the patient as culturally different from yourself. You can use the CFI profitably in any setting because "cultural" accounts of why people get ill and why people return to health occur not only in immigrant communities but in all communities. A person whom you believe to share your own cultural account of illness and health often has a very different understanding of why people become ill and how they can become well. Furthermore, the CFI is the most patient-centered portion of DSM-5, and using it particularizes the diagnostic process. The CFI is not a scored system of symptoms but rather a series of prompts to help you assess how a patient understands his distress, its etiology, its treatment, and prognosis. I include an operationalized version of the CFI in Chapter 11 of this book, but additional information is available in DSM-5 itself. Online, at www.psychiatry.org/dsm5, you can find alternative versions of the CFI and supplementary modules.

Conclusion

By introducing dimensions, the authors of DSM-5 are trying to increase the accuracy of current diagnoses while reducing the number of diagnoses ascribed to each patient. At the same time, they hope the clinical use of dimensions will identify relationships between disorders that were separated in strictly categorical diagnostic systems, such as DSM-IV. For example, although major depressive disorder and alcohol use disorder are known to be associated with each other, the precise nature of their association is unclear. To return to the situation with which this chapter began, the careful use of dimensions may help identify a subset of people whose depression is etiologically connected to their panic in a previously unknown fashion. In this way, a dimensional diagnostic system could spur research by identifying unknown connections or by explaining associations that are not yet understood.

Before the arrival of DSM-5, its authors insisted that dimensions were the signal advance of DSM-5, and critics described the introduction of dimensions as DSM-5's chief flaw. Critics argued that dimensions encourage interviewers to measure rather than to interpret symptoms. Dimensions, they contended, are more useful for researchers than for clinicians (Phillips et al. 2012c).

As a compromise, the authors of DSM-5 ultimately elected to introduce dimensions in a subtle fashion, chiefly for screening tools and rating systems. They piloted, but did not adopt, dimensional approaches to personality disorders. However, they insist that dimensions remain the future of psychiatric diagnostic systems. Indeed, if you look at Chapter 13, "Alternative Diagnostic Systems and Rating Scales," you can see that the concept of dimensions has support from both psychoanalysts and neuroscientists. For now, practitioners will ultimately decide the impact of DSM-5's dimensional tools by how widely and how well they employ them in clinical practice.

Chapter 5

Key Changes in DSM-5

DSM-5 serves as a bridge from the current diagnostic system, which is based on symptom categories, to a future diagnostic system based on disturbances in specific, interconnected circuits of the brain (Kupfer and Regier 2011). As discussed in Chapter 4, "Adventures in Dimensions," dimensions are the essential supports in this bridge, but interviewers also need to know about other changes in DSM-5. The authors of DSM-5 refined the diagnostic criteria for all of the included diagnoses and altered the presentation of diagnoses. In this chapter, I review how these DSM-5 changes alter the diagnostic interview by examining cases involving four common diagnoses. In the final section of this chapter, I discuss the end of the multiaxial assessment system and describe how DSM-5 renews attention to developmental processes in its diagnostic categories.

Major Depressive Disorder

Ruth is a 56-year-old teacher with no past psychiatric history who reports that for 3 weeks she has been hearing the voice of her deceased husband telling her that he misses her. He died of a heart attack while they were attending the wedding of one of their three children. Ruth and her husband had enjoyed a close relationship, and they had been looking forward to celebrating their thirtieth anniversary later in the year. Although her husband had high cholesterol and hypertension, Ruth was surprised by his death and worries that she "should have seen it coming and saved him." She feels guilty about his death, especially at night, when she is unable to sleep more than a couple of hours. She denies thoughts of suicide, but wonders frequently if her life is still worth living. She describes her mood as down, reports poor energy, and appears fatigued. She admits that her appetite is decreased and shrugs her shoulders when asked if she has lost weight. She says she has been attending to her grieving family and returned to work last week without difficulty, but feels disinterested. Ruth denies any previous depressive, hypomanic, or manic episodes and drinks alcohol only at social events.

The main criteria for a major depressive disorder have not changed substantially between DSM-IV (and DSM-IV-TR) and DSM-5. An episode is still defined by the presence of five or more of the following symptoms during the same 2-week period: depressed mood, anhedonia, significant weight loss or weight gain, insomnia or hypersomnia, psychomotor agitation or retardation, fatigue or loss of energy, feelings of worthlessness or excessive guilt, diminished concentration, and recurrent thoughts of death or suicide. In DSM-5, as in DSM-IV, an episode must include depressed mood or anhedonia, cause significant distress, and not be caused by substance use or another medical condition.

So what is different? Ruth's presentation demonstrates two important differences. First, Ruth clearly associates her depression with the death of her husband. In DSM-IV, her presentation might not meet criteria for a major depressive episode because it could be considered bereavement, which is itself a kind of culturally conditioned illness. This exclusion is removed in DSM-5, so Ruth's presentation meets the criteria for major depressive disorder, single episode. Second, the specifiers for her diagnosis are different in DSM-5. An episode of depression can now be specified as being with psychotic features but as not being severe. In DSM-IV, the presence of psychotic symptoms necessarily meant the episode was severe. Because Ruth is still working and attending to her family, her episode could be classified as moderate using DSM-5, but with psychotic features because she is hearing the voice of her deceased husband.

Schizophrenia

Woo-jin is a 33-year-old public policy graduate student who enrolled at a local university 9 months ago. During his first semester, he kept to himself. His grades were mediocre, so the college assigned him a tutor for the second semester. Woo-jin has attended tutoring sessions only sporadically, and when he arrives, he is often late and poorly groomed. Although he says little, when he does speak, it is often about how his classmates conspire against him. When you evaluate him with the assistance of an interpreter and ask for evidence of this conspiracy, he alludes to information he received from course readings and a podcast. He shows you a page from a social networking site on his smartphone as evidence and becomes upset as he discusses it, but all you can see are invitations to lectures and messages from study partners. As he discusses his concerns, you find it progressively harder to understand him because he shifts from one topic to another without a clear connection. When you ask about his grades, he admits they are even worse this semester, but blames the government for his grades. When you ask if the situation has gotten so bad that he wants to return to his home country, he shrugs his shoulders and admits that his own government is conspiring against him as well. He shakes his head when you ask if he is depressed, but he exhibits a flat affect and often appears to be engaged in an internal conversation.

The essential criteria for schizophrenia and the time course remain the same in DSM-5 as in DSM-IV. For these criteria to be met, a person must have been experiencing continuous signs of disturbance for at least 6 months and two or more of the following symptoms for at least 1 month: delusions, hallucinations, disorganized speech, grossly abnormal psychomotor behavior, and negative symptoms. To qualify, disturbances must include at least one of these core symptoms: delusions, hallucinations, and disorganized speech. When you are interviewing a patient, remember that a belief that is idiosyncratic is not necessarily delusional. DSM-5 clearly notes that in "some cultures, visual or auditory hallucinations with a religious content…are a normal part of religious experience" (American Psychiatric Association 2013, p. 103). According to DSM-5, whenever a patient has a different cultural, religious, or linguistic background from the interviewer, diagnostic care must be taken to avoid pathologizing difference. Indeed, the manual has specific advice for the diagnostic interview, encouraging interviewers struggling to distinguish between odd and psychotic beliefs to assess if seemingly odd beliefs are grounded in reality, linked to an external stimulus, coherent and goal-directed, and communicated with an appropriate range of affective, motor, and verbal behavior. If a belief meets all of these criteria, it is less likely to be a psychotic belief. If you are still struggling to determine whether a belief is delusional, consider using the Cultural Formulation Interview, which is discussed in Chapter 11, "Selected DSM-5 Assessment Measures." In this way, DSM-5 renews attention to cultural variations and strives to distinguish the normal, but unfamiliar, from the frankly psychotic.

In addition, the authors of DSM-5 removed several familiar diagnostic subtypes. In DSM-IV, a person with Woo-jin's presentation would be categorized as having paranoid schizophrenia. In DSM-5, the types of schizophrenia have been eliminated. According to researchers, schizophrenia remains a heterogeneous disorder, but DSM-IV's subtypes suggested a degree of division between subtypes on the basis of symptoms that was not borne out in clinical practice. A person with schizophrenia can still be diagnosed with a specific course (first or multiple episodes, partial or full remission, continuous, or acute episode) that can now be described either as having prominent negative features or as occurring with catatonia, but the task of trying to distinguish between paranoid and disorganized schizophrenia has been eliminated in DSM-5. Finally, the dimensional system allows for acknowledgment of concomitant disturbances in cognition, depression, and mania in a person diagnosed with schizophrenia using the Clinician-Rated Dimensions of Psychosis Symptom Severity, included in Chapter 11.

Alcohol Use Disorder

Kagiso is a 47-year-old emergency room physician who began drinking socially during medical school. Her alcohol use has gradually escalated over the last two decades, and she "cannot recall" the last time she went a day without at least three drinks. She has missed several emergency department shifts because she was too intoxicated to attend. Over the last 2 years, she has tried to control her drinking by having two drinks before her shifts in the emergency department and "a few more" after work. Over the last 6 months, several nurses have reported her for odd medical decisions. Yesterday, a colleague discovered her drinking in a call room. She was told to enter a residential impaired physician program or risk having her employment terminated. During the admission evaluation to a residential treatment facility, Kagiso acknowledges that she would like to stop drinking, admitting that alcohol contributed to the dissolution of her marriage but that she has been unable to reduce her alcohol intake. When she last tried to, she became tremulous and sweaty approximately 6 hours after her last drink and she began drinking again for fear she would suffer a seizure.

In DSM-5, substances of abuse are grouped into nine classes—alcohol; caffeine; cannabis; hallucinogens (which include PCP [phencyclidine], LSD [lysergic acid diethylamide], and MDMA [3,4-methylenedioxymethamphetamine]); inhalants; opioids; sedatives, hypnotics, and anxiolytics; stimulants (which include amphetamine and cocaine); and tobacco—but similar criteria are used to describe their abuse. The authors explain this approach by noting that although these substances have different effects, they all activate the brain's reward system. On this basis, the authors of DSM-5 included gambling disorder in the same category as substance use disorders (a category termed *substance-related and addictive disorders*), because they found sufficient evidence for a common neural pathway: the activation of the brain's reward system. This is a conceptual change and, in the case of gambling disorder, a novel diagnosis for DSM-5—one that signals the authors' intent to eventually organize all mental disorders according to their underlying pathology.

What the authors did not retain was the DSM-IV distinction between substance abuse and substance dependence. According to DSM-IV, an individual was diagnosed with substance dependence rather than substance abuse based on tolerance, withdrawal, use of a substance in larger amounts or over a longer period than was intended, and a desire to quit or unsuccessful attempts to reduce use (American Psychiatric Association 2000, p. 197). The authors of DSM-5 were concerned that the substance dependence criteria could not distinguish between someone with pharmacological dependence, tolerance, and withdrawal—an expected consequence in someone prescribed maintenance doses of, say, methadone or a benzodiazepine—and someone who had developed physiological dependence from abusing substances. In other words, they believed that earlier DSM versions did not sufficiently consider the intent of a person who used a potentially abusive substance. This change in DSM-5 corrects a problem seen often in clinical practice. A psychiatrist might diagnose a patient as having "iatrogenic opiate dependence with physiological dependence," a diagnosis that was not in DSM-IV but that nevertheless characterized clearly a patient's substance use. DSM-5 resolves that problem by removing the various substance dependence categories.

Instead, DSM-5 provides use, intoxication, and withdrawal categories, along with substance-induced categories of mental disorders. Although the criteria are distinct for each substance, they follow the general pattern established for alcohol. Diagnosis of an alcohol use disorder requires at least two of the following symptoms in a 12-month period: tolerance; withdrawal; drinking more alcohol or drinking for a longer period than intended; failed attempts to reduce or cease use; spending a significant amount of time obtaining or recovering from alcohol; craving alcohol; recurrent use resulting in failure to fulfill major role obligations; continued use despite its association with interpersonal problems; reducing or giving up important social, occupational, or recreational activities because of the alcohol use; recurrent use in situations that are physically hazardous; and continued use despite awareness that the alcohol causes or exacerbates a physical or psychological problem.

Kagiso's presentation clearly meets the criteria for an alcohol use disorder. In addition, it would be appropriate to use two specifiers to better characterize her diagnosis. Because she has been admitted to a residential treatment facility, her course would be described as "in a controlled environment" under the DSM-5 rubric. Because she endorses four or more of the criteria, her diagnosis would be described as severe.

Narcissistic Personality Disorder

Keith is a 33-year-old assistant professor who has just been denied tenure despite having written what he calls "the best dissertation in my field in the last century." After receiving notice that he would not receive tenure, Keith angrily quit his position. He has sought legal counsel to sue his university, but says, "None of the attorneys I have contacted is sufficiently well trained to represent me," insisting that they would need a doctorate in his own field as well as a legal degree "from a top-five research university" to grasp his situation. You are meeting with Keith because an attorney suggested you could assist him in crafting an appropriate strategy. Keith begins the meeting by asking about your training and asking for copies "of your 10 most important papers." He denies manic, depressive, and psychotic symptoms, and insists that his only problem is that "other people cannot understand me." He was twice engaged but never married because "they were not distinguished enough." When asked if he has close friends, he names several historical figures, saying, "Those are the kind of people whom I see as my peers." When asked about his colleagues at the university, he complains that they were too "envious of me to be true peers."

In DSM-5, personality disorders can be diagnosed by one of two systems. The first system is a categorical system familiar to any interviewer experienced with DSM-IV. This system is in the main text of DSM-5 and is endorsed for regular clinical use. (It is also the system used in Chapters 3 and 6 of this book.) The second system is a dimensional system. This system is the "Emerging Measures and Models" of DSM-5 and is endorsed for research use. We can consider Keith's presentation using both systems.

In the categorical model endorsed for clinical work, Keith's presentation clearly meets the criteria for narcissistic personality disorder. He endorses at least five of the enumerated manifestations of this personality disorder. All nine of the manifestations remain the same between DSM-IV and DSM-5. The diagnosis remains without exclusion criteria.

What has changed? DSM-5 still lists 10 specific personality disorders and the symptomatic manifestations of each disorder remain the same. The general definition of a personality disorder as "an enduring pattern of inner experience and behavior that deviates markedly from the expectations of the individual's culture" (American Psychiatric Association, 2013, p. 645) is also unchanged. The personality disorders are still organized into Cluster A, for people who often appear odd or eccentric; Cluster B, for people who often appear dramatic, emotional, or erratic; and Cluster C, for people who often appear anxious or fearful.

In short, DSM-5 endorses a diagnostic system for clinical use in which personality disorders are organized based on appearances. The authors acknowledge that even when used properly, their current categorical system often leads to the diagnosis of multiple personality disorders in the same person and widespread use of the unspecified personality disorder diagnosis.

To address these problems, DSM-5 characterizes a dimensional approach, based on underlying psychological traits, as the future way to identify personality disorders. The dimensional model was deemed not ready for DSM-5, but it may very well be in DSM-5.1, so we review it here.

The dimensional approach is a remarkable change in the categorical features and conceptualization of personality disorders. On a practical level, the DSM-5 personality disorder work group removed four personality disorders—paranoid, schizoid, histrionic, and dependent—after determining that they lacked sufficient evidence for their utility and validity.

The DSM-5 work group found sufficient evidence to support the retention of only six categorical DSM-5 personality disorders—antisocial, avoidant, borderline, narcissistic, obsessive-compulsive, and schizotypal—and refined their diagnostic criteria thoroughly. In general, the work group reduced attention to behavior in the categorical diagnoses of personality disorders in favor of assessing functional impairments. In short, they encourage diagnosing a personality disorder only when a person has an impaired ability to establish a coherent identity, to be self-directed, to develop empathy for others, and to develop reciprocal relationships. You still identify pathological personality traits, but only after first establishing whether the patient has impairment in self-functioning and interpersonal functioning.

The authors of DSM-5 designed this dimensional approach to limit the diagnosis of personality disorders to those with the strongest evidence base, to reduce the diagnosis of multiple personality disorders in a single person, and to remove the diagnosis of personality disorder not otherwise specified. With the dimensional model, you can diagnose one of the six personality disorders named above and specify additional traits for each, or you can use a new diagnosis, personality disorder—trait specified, to indicate the presence of specific traits that do not reach the level of a particular diagnosis.

Keith's example illustrates several of these changes. In the categorical model retained in DSM-5, an arbitrary number of personality traits led to a diagnosis. In DSM-5's proposed dimensional model, the diagnosis of narcissistic personality disorder begins with impairments in self-functioning and interpersonal functioning. To meet the criteria, a patient must have impairment in self-functioning as indicated either by excessive reference to others for self-definition and self-esteem or by goal setting based on gaining approval from others. She must also have impairment in interpersonal functioning as indicated by a lack of empathy or an inability to experience emotionally intimate relationships with others. Unlike in earlier models of personality disorders, these functional impairments are common to all personality disorders. If a patient endorses these impairments in self-functioning and interpersonal functioning, the interviewer is prompted to characterize which pathological personality traits are present. I model this in Chapter 12, "Dimensional Diagnosis of Personality Disorders." If we use this model to consider Keith's presentation, the pathological personality traits are grandiosity and attention seeking.

Grandiosity and attention seeking are what the DSM-5 dimensional model calls "facets" of antagonism, one of the Five Factors used as an organizing principle for personality disorder diagnoses. In the literature, *Five-Factor Model* usually refers to the adaptive personality traits of neuroticism, extraversion, agreeableness, conscientiousness, and openness to experience (Digman 1990). Because the DSM-5 work group built these diagnostic criteria from a deficit-based rather than a strength-based model, they organized personality disorders around five companion maladaptive traits: negative affectivity, detachment, antagonism, disinhibition, and psychoticism. The authors found compelling evidence for these five maladaptive traits as stable and predictive of problems in self-functioning and interpersonal functioning. In addition, they identified "facets" for each of these five maladaptive traits. In total, DSM-5 enumerates 25 facets organized into five domains for each of the maladaptive traits listed above. The Five-Factor Model replaces the so-called cluster model of categorical versions, in which personality disorders are organized into Cluster A, B, and C disorders.

The presence of grandiosity and attention seeking is necessary but not sufficient for a diagnosis of narcissistic personality disorder in the dimensional model. To make the diagnosis, you need to find evidence of impairment in self-functioning and interpersonal functioning. The authors of DSM-5 provide a 5-point scale, ranging from 0 (little or no impairment) to 4 (extreme impairment), that they call the *Level of Personality Functioning Scale,* which is included in Chapter 12 of this guidebook. This scale is an example of a dimensional assessment directly incorporated into diagnostic criteria in an effort to diagnose patients only when the diagnosis has the greatest predictive power of dysfunction. Based on their analysis of the data, the DSM-5 authors concluded that the presence of personality traits is most meaningful when a patient is experiencing profound impairment in self-functioning and interpersonal functioning. In the instance of Keith, even this brief sketch suggests that his narcissistic traits are interfering, at the least, with his work and his romantic life. After a thorough assessment, his level of impairment would likely be scored as 4 (Extreme Impairment) on the Level of Personality Functioning Scale.

However, if Keith had presented with self-functioning and interpersonal functioning impairments sufficient to meet criteria for a personality disorder but had not exhibited the specific traits associated with a named personality disorder, he would have been diagnosed with a personality disorder—trait specified in the dimensional model. Using the five domains named above, you could conduct a personality overview sufficient to specify a trait and make the diagnosis. If doing so would guide your diagnosis and treatment, you could alternatively use the 25 trait facets to create a personality profile in addition to the diagnosis. This process, using the Personality Trait Rating Form, is described in Chapter 12.

In reading about it, this process likely seems confusing. Its merit is that it limits named personality disorders to those with the greatest validity and utility, requires evidence of serious impairment in self-functioning and interpersonal functioning, and implicitly defines healthy personality functioning, all while allowing you to make a diagnosis when evaluating someone with such impairments even if all the criteria for a specific diagnosis are not met. The authors of DSM-5 conceive of the dimensional diagnosis of a personality disorder as occurring in a stepwise process, beginning with determining whether a patient's presentation meets criteria for a personality disorder. This determination is based on 1) the extent to which she experiences impairments in self-functioning and interpersonal functioning and 2) the extent to which she meets criteria for one of the six named personality disorders or, finally, for personality disorder—trait specified, listing whichever of the five maladaptive traits (negative affectivity, detachment, antagonism, disinhibition, and psychoticism) the patient expresses. These changes in the diagnostic process for personality disorders are an attempt to use the best evidence available, while being flexible enough for clinical practice, and are reflected in the operationalized criteria presented in Chapter 12 of this pocket guide.

Reordering of Disorders

In addition to making various categorical changes, some of which I discussed above, the authors of DSM-5 rearranged the sequence of disorders by eliminating the multiaxial system and by integrating developmental and temperamental considerations into the organization of DSM-5.

Although previous DSM editions did not require the use of the multiaxial system, it was widely adopted in clinical practice. Since its introduction in DSM-III, a generation of practitioners have documented primary mental disorders on Axis I;

mental retardation, personality disorders, and characteristic defense mechanisms on Axis II; general medical conditions that contribute to mental distress on Axis III; psychosocial problems on Axis IV; and the Global Assessment of Functioning scale score on Axis V. By presenting a person's diagnoses along the multiaxial system, clinicians drew attention to the multiplicity of factors involved in mental distress. In a categorical diagnostic system that explicitly avoids discussing the etiology of mental distress, the resulting diagnoses are implicitly divided by putative etiology, with "real" mental illnesses on Axis I, character pathology on Axis II, medical illnesses on Axis III, and social problems on Axis IV. In this respect, a multiaxial diagnosis was the perplexing result of a diagnostic interview from a manual that maintained an intentional silence about etiology.

Because the authors of DSM-5 preserved the atheoretical and categorical principles of previous editions, they have logically abandoned the multiaxial system. Instead, the result of a DSM-5 diagnostic interview is now a diagnosis, or several diagnoses, when indicated, all listed together. The authors of DSM-5 have collapsed Axes I through III into a single diagnostic list that includes diagnoses previously listed on Axes I and II, along with nonpsychiatric medical conditions that significantly contribute to a person's mental disorder. Because Axis III often became a list of all the medical problems a person had ever experienced, it was not uncommon for a scrupulous trainee to list, for instance, an arm broken in adolescence and fully healed as one of the admission diagnoses of a middle-aged man. The broken arm was listed even though it had no discernible effect on his presenting mental distress. You do not need to list a historical or chronic medical condition on the DSM-5 diagnostic list unless it alters your interpretation or treatment of a person's mental disorder.

In addition, the multiaxial system consisted of fundamentally different categories—well-structured diagnoses on Axes I through III, an unstructured list of psychosocial problems on Axis IV, and a functional assessment on Axis V—and thus implicitly confused diagnoses and functional assessments. Axes IV and V were both widely misused, either as an unstructured list of psychosocial problems in the case of Axis IV, or as crude estimates of illness severity to ensure insurance approval in the case of Axis V. In place of Axis IV, DSM-5 uses the more formal V and Z codes of ICD-9 and ICD-10, respectively (World Health Organization 1992) to list psychosocial and environmental problems that alter the diagnosis, treatment, and prognosis of a person's mental disorder. Instead of Axis V, which conflated symptom severity and functional impairment (Goldman et al. 1992), DSM-5 uses the World Health Organization Disability Assessment Schedule 2.0 (WHODAS 2.0; World Health Organization 2010), which is a well-validated assessment of functioning on six subscales. A list of ICD-9-CM V codes and ICD-10-CM Z codes and information about WHODAS 2.0 can be found in Chapters 6 and 11, respectively.

In previous DSM versions, disorders were grouped by their usual age at onset: during infancy, childhood, adolescence, or adulthood. In contrast, the authors of DSM-5 organized disorders by common phenomenology and pathology rather than by age at onset. As a result, disorders that are most often diagnosed in children, such as separation anxiety disorder or pica, are found alongside their respective pathological neighbors—in these cases, anxiety disorders and feeding and eating disorders, respectively. In addition, the DSM-5 criteria for a condition most commonly diagnosed in adults, such as an anxiety disorder or depressive disorder, include additional information about how development influences the onset, presentation, and course of the disorder. The goal is to show how a person might experience a mental disorder differently during various developmental stages. To further emphasize a developmental perspective, the authors of DSM-5 present pathological categories roughly in the order in which they present, beginning with neurodevelopmental disorders and ending with paraphilic disorders.

The authors of DSM-5 also group the disorder categories by the presence of either internalizing or externalizing factors. Disorders associated with internalizing factors, such as depressive disorders and anxiety disorders, are presented earlier in DSM-5. They are followed by disorders associated with externalizing factors, such as antisocial and elimination disorders, because the authors implicitly point to future editions in which psychiatric disorders will likely be organized by their underlying dysfunction. In a similar way, DSM-5 includes the etiology for several neurocognitive disorders. As the causes of mental disorders are identified, I anticipate that future versions of DSM will similarly identify them in the diagnostic criteria.

Finally, DSM-5 replaces the "not otherwise specified" (NOS) classification with "other specified" and "unspecified." DSM-IV's NOS diagnosis allowed a clinician to initiate treatment for a patient whose presentation was not consistent with a more specific diagnosis. The heterogeneity of this category discouraged research, frustrated epidemiology, and diminished the clinical utility of diagnoses (Fairburn and Bohn 2005). In at least some situations, NOS diagnoses were found to be less stable over time when compared with diagnoses that met the more specific criteria (Rondeau et al. 2011), decreasing their reliability and validity.

The "unspecified" and "other specified" criteria are found in each chapter of DSM-5 and provide more details than the comparable NOS sections in DSM-IV. In general, interviewers are advised to consider "unspecified" diagnoses when a person experiences symptoms characteristic of a mental disorder that cause clinically significant distress but do not meet full criteria for a named diagnosis. If an interviewer wishes to communicate the specific reason a person does not meet criteria, the interviewer is encouraged to use the "other specified" diagnosis. For example, a person who experiences persistent auditory hallucinations in the absence of other features of schizophrenia would be diagnosed with other specified schizophrenia spectrum and other psychotic disorder (persistent auditory hallucinations).

Conclusion

The authors of DSM-5 revised the diagnostic criteria and the conceptualization of every diagnosis to reflect recent advances. In this chapter, I demonstrated how the criteria and the conceptualization have changed for each of four diagnoses, selected for discussion because of their importance in clinical practice. Considering these four representative diagnoses illustrates the difficult task faced by the authors of DSM-5 to use the best available data while creating useful diagnostic criteria. As a clinician and teacher, I find that the major depressive disorder, schizophrenia, and alcohol use disorder criteria strike the correct balance, by removing subtypes and qualifiers that were often difficult to distinguish. At this point, I find the categorical personality disorder criteria inadequate and the dimensional personality disorder criteria easier to appreciate than to put into practice.

However, this change is also the most exciting to me, because it better reflects the complexity of persons in distress. Indeed, it serves as a model for the operationalized version of the diagnostic exam in Chapter 6, where you ask a few screening questions and then establish impairment before asking more specific criteria. By all accounts, some version of this is the future of psychiatric diagnosis. If, at various points in the last two centuries, our diagnostic systems were designed for the asylum, the battlefield, the outpatient clinic, or the research university (e.g., Grob 1991; Houts 2000), the diagnostic system of the future will likely be designed for the mental health practitioner as consultant. In a world with a limited number of mental health providers, we will probably focus on diagnosing and initiating treatment. In the following chapter, I offer one way to do so.

SECTION II

Chapter 6

The DSM-5
Diagnostic Interview

In Chapter 3, "The 30-Minute Diagnostic Interview," I outlined a diagnostic interview that included a screening question for each of the DSM-5 categories of mental disorders. If a person answers affirmatively to one of those questions, what do you do? In this chapter, I demonstrate how the screening questions are the avenues of the psychiatric diagnostic interview. A good interviewer skillfully travels these avenues with a patient and, when possible, reaches a specific and accurate diagnosis along the way.

This chapter follows the order of DSM-5 disorders, beginning with neurodevelopmental disorders. For each category of DSM-5 diagnoses presented, whether bipolar disorders or elimination disorders, the section begins with one or more screening questions from the model interview presented in Chapter 3. After the screening questions, there are follow-up questions. If the follow-up questions include a measure of impairment or a measure of time, these measures are a required part of the subsequent diagnostic criteria. By putting follow-up questions before the additional symptom questions in the diagnostic criteria, I am attempting to make the interview more efficient and precise while reserving full diagnosis of a mental disorder for a person who is impaired by his experiences.

The screening and follow-up questions are followed by the diagnostic criteria. When the diagnostic criteria are to be elicited by the interviewer, I offer italicized prompts for the relevant symptom. I structured these questions so that an affirmative answer meets the criteria for that symptom. When the diagnostic criteria are observed rather than elicited, as in the case of disorganized speech or psychomotor retardation or autonomic hyperactivity, they are listed as instructions to the interviewer, set in roman type. The minimum number of symptoms necessary to reach a particular diagnosis is underlined.

Questions specifically included for children and adolescents are shaded. Of course, I do not list all the possible questions that can be used to elicit a relevant symptom, but these questions are specifically designed to follow DSM-5. To make the diagnostic process as clear as possible, I have included negative criteria for a DSM-5 diagnosis under the heading "Exclusion." For example, DSM-5 observes that a person's presentation does not meet criteria for schizophrenia if he experiences psychotic symptoms only as the direct physiological effect of a substance. These exclusion criteria usually do not require you to ask a specific question, but instead depend on the history you elicit. The most common subtypes, specifiers, and severity measures are listed under the heading "Modifiers."

In the interest of brevity, this guide includes diagnostic questions for the most common DSM-5 disorders. The idea is to focus on learning the diagnostic criteria for the paradigmatic disorders in each section before exploring the related diagnoses—that is, to know the main streets of DSM-5 before learning its side streets.

In this book, the side streets are labeled as "alternatives," a term that is not used in DSM-5. These alternatives include only related diagnoses from the same DSM-5 chapter. For example, adjustment disorder is listed as an alternative to post-traumatic stress disorder (PTSD), because they are grouped together in DSM-5. In contrast, traumatic brain injury and other diagnoses listed in the differential diagnosis for PTSD are not in the "alternatives" section for PTSD, because they are found in different sections of DSM-5. For each diagnosis listed in "alternatives," the essential diagnostic criteria are included and the interviewer is referred to the corresponding pages in DSM-5 to read the diagnostic criteria and associated material in detail.

Although this guide includes all the diagnoses within DSM-5, it eliminates repetitive criteria, especially for the various mental disorders associated with another medical condition or substance-induced mental disorders, in which, broadly, the symptoms of a disorder are present as a direct effect of another medical condition or the use of a substance.

As this overview suggests, this book is no substitute for DSM-5 but serves as a practical diagnostic tool, an operationalized version of DSM-5—the equivalent of the sketched version of a city street that a GPS device displays, rather than the detailed portrait of each side street. This book will help you reach your destination in a timely fashion but without the rich detail of DSM-5. In the abstract, this diagnostic interview process may sound confusing; however, once you start with a common diagnosis (say, bipolar disorder), read through the interview material once, and practice it a few times, the organization should become clear.

Neurodevelopmental Disorders

DSM-5 pp. 31–86

Screening questions for a person (or caregiver): *Did you have any behavioral or learning problems during your early childhood? When you started school, did you have trouble relating socially or keeping up academically with your classmates because of behavioral or learning problems?*

    If yes, ask: *Do you have trouble concentrating or struggle with being impulsive or hyperactive? Do you have difficulty communicating with other people or in social interactions? Are there specific bothersome behaviors that you do frequently and find hard to control? Do you struggle to learn, more than your classmates do?*

- If deficits in intellectual functioning or specific academic skills predominate, proceed to intellectual disability (intellectual developmental disorder) criteria.
- If deficits in social interactions or impairing motor behaviors predominate, proceed to autism spectrum disorder criteria.
- If inattention, hyperactivity, or impulsivity predominate, proceed to attention-deficit/hyperactivity disorder criteria.

1. Intellectual Disability (Intellectual Developmental Disorder)

   a. Inclusion: Requires intellectual deficits, beginning during the developmental period, that impair adaptive function as manifested by <u>both</u> of the following symptoms.

      i. Deficits in intellectual functions, such as reasoning, problem solving, planning, abstract thinking, judgment, academic learning, and experiential learning. Must be confirmed by both clinical assessment and individualized, standardized intelligence testing.

ii. Impaired adaptive functioning, normalized for developmental and sociocultural standards, which restricts participation and performance in one or more aspects of daily life activities. The limitations result in the need for ongoing support at school, at work, or for independent life.

b. Modifiers

   i. Severity (see DSM-5, pp. 34–36, Table 1)

   • Mild
   • Moderate
   • Severe
   • Profound

c. Alternatives

   i. If a person younger than 5 years fails to meet expected developmental milestones in several areas of intellectual functioning and is unable to undergo systematic assessments of intellectual functioning, consider global developmental delay (see DSM-5, p. 41). This diagnosis requires eventual reassessment.

   ii. If a person older than 5 years exhibits intellectual disability that cannot be well characterized because of associated sensory or physical impairments, consider unspecified intellectual disability (see DSM-5, p. 41). This diagnosis should be used only in exceptional circumstances and requires eventual reassessment.

   iii. If a person has persistent difficulties in the acquisition and use of language (spoken, written, sign, or other modalities) that begin in the early developmental period and result in substantial functional limitations, consider the diagnosis of language disorder (full criteria are available in DSM-5, p. 42). Language disorder occurs as a primary impairment or may coexist with other disorders. This diagnosis should not be used if the language difficulties are better explained by hearing or sensory impairment, intellectual disability, or global developmental delay or are caused by another medical or neurological condition.

   iv. If a person has persistent difficulties in speech sound production that interfere with speech intelligibility or prevent verbal communication of messages, consider speech sound disorder (full criteria are available in DSM-5, p. 44). The symptoms must be present in the early developmental period and result in limitations in effective communication, social participation, academic achievement, and occupational performance, individually or in any combination. Speech sound disorder occurs as a primary impairment or coexists with other disorders or congenital or acquired conditions. This diagnosis should not be used if the speech sound difficulties are due to congenital or acquired medical or neurological conditions.

v. If a person has marked and frequent disturbances in the fluency and time patterning of speech that are inappropriate for the person's age and language skills, consider childhood-onset fluency disorder (stuttering) (full criteria are available in DSM-5, pp. 45–46). Symptoms must begin in the early developmental period. The disturbance must cause anxiety about speaking or the ability to communicate effectively. This disorder can coexist with other disorders. However, the diagnosis should not be used if the disorder is attributable to a speech-motor or sensory deficit, is due to another medical or neurological condition, or is better explained by another mental disorder.

vi. If a person has persistent difficulties in the social use of verbal and nonverbal communication that functionally limit effective communication, social participation, social relationships, academic achievement, or occupational performance, consider social (pragmatic) communication disorder (full criteria are available in DSM-5, pp. 47–48). Symptoms begin during the early developmental period. The disorder can coexist with other disorders. However, this diagnosis should not be used if the symptoms are better explained by intellectual disability, global developmental delay, or another mental disorder or are due to another medical or neurological condition.

vii. If a person has symptoms of a communication disorder that cause clinically significant distress or impairment but do not meet the full criteria for a communication disorder or another neurodevelopmental disorder, consider unspecified communication disorder (see DSM-5, p. 49).

    viii. If a person has persistent difficulties in learning and using academic skills that begin during school-age years and eventually result in significant interference with academic or occupational performance, consider specific learning disorder (full criteria, along with severity ratings, are available in DSM-5, pp. 66–68). To meet criteria, the current skills must be well below the average range for the person's age, gender, cultural group, and level of education. The symptoms must not be better accounted for by another intellectual, medical, mental, neurological, or sensory disorder.

2. Autism Spectrum Disorder

    a. Inclusion: Requires persistent deficits in social communication and social interaction, across multiple contexts, that are present in the early developmental period but that may not be manifest until social demands exceed limited capacities, and that cause clinically significant impairment in functioning. The disorder is marked by, for example, <u>all</u> of the following persistent deficits in social communication and interaction.

        i. Deficits in social-emotional reciprocity: *When you meet someone, how do you introduce yourself? Do you find it hard to greet another person? Do you find it hard to share your interests, thoughts, and feelings with other people? Do you dislike to hear about what other people are interested in or how they feel?*

        ii. Deficits in nonverbal communicative behaviors used for social interaction; these are usually observed by the interviewer and range from poorly integrated verbal and nonverbal communication, through abnormalities in eye contact and body language, or deficits in understanding and use of nonverbal communication, to total lack of facial expression or gestures.

        iii. Deficits in developing and maintaining relationships: *Are you disinterested in other people? Are you unable to engage in imaginative play with other people? Do you find it difficult to make new friends? When the situation around you changes, do you find it hard to adjust your own behavior in response?*

b. Inclusion: In addition, the diagnosis requires at least <u>two</u> of the following signs of restricted, repetitive patterns of behavior, interests, or activities.

   i. Stereotyped or repetitive speech, motor movements, or use of objects, such as simple motor stereotypies, echolalia, repetitive use of objects, or idiosyncratic phrases.

   ii. Insistence on sameness and excessive adherence to routines or avoidance of change: *Do you have any special routines or patterns of behavior? What happens when you cannot follow these routines or engage in these behaviors? Do you struggle to change?*

   iii. Restricted interests of abnormal intensity or focus: *Do you intensely focus upon, or find yourself very interested in, just a few things?*

   iv. Hyper- or hyporeactivity to sensory input: *How do you experience something that is painful? Something hot? Something cold? Are there particular sounds, textures, or smells to which you respond strongly? Do you find yourself fascinated with lights or spinning objects?*

c. Modifiers

   i. Specifiers

   • With (or without) accompanying intellectual impairment
   • With (or without) accompanying language impairment
   • Associated with a known medical or genetic condition or environmental factor
   • Associated with another neurodevelopmental, mental, or behavioral disorder
   • With catatonia

   ii. Severity is coded separately for the social communication impairments and for the restricted, repetitive patterns of behavior.

   • Level 1: Requiring support
   • Level 2: Requiring substantial support
   • Level 3: Requiring very substantial support

d. Alternatives

   i. If a person exhibits coordinated motor performance substantially below expected levels, which significantly interferes with activities of daily living or academic achievement and which began in the early developmental period, consider developmental coordination disorder (full criteria are in DSM-5, p. 74). Examples include clumsiness, as well as slow and inaccurate performance of motor skills. The disturbance cannot be due to another medical or neurological condition or be better explained by another mental disorder.

ii. If a person exhibits repetitive, seemingly driven, yet apparently purposeless motor behavior, such as hand shaking or waving, body rocking, head banging, or self-biting, consider stereotypic movement disorder (full criteria are in DSM-5, pp. 77–78). The motor disturbance causes clinically significant distress or impairment. The motor behavior is not due to the direct physiological effects of a substance or a general medical condition and is not better explained by the symptoms of another mental disorder.

iii. A tic is a sudden, rapid, recurrent, nonrhythmic motor movement or vocalization. If a person experiences both motor and vocal tics beginning before age 18 years, consider Tourette's disorder (full criteria are in DSM-5, p. 81). The tics may wax and wane in frequency but must persist for at least 1 year after onset. The tics cannot be due to the direct physiological effects of another medical condition or a substance.

iv. If a person experiences either motor or vocal tics, but not both, during his illness, and has never met criteria for Tourette's disorder, consider persistent (chronic) motor or vocal tic disorder (full criteria are in DSM-5, p. 81). The onset is before age 18 years, and the tics may wax and wane in frequency but must have persisted for more than 1 year since their onset.

v.   If a person experiences motor and/or vocal tics for at least 1 year, beginning before age 18 years, and the tics are not due to the direct physiological consequences of a substance or another medical condition, and he has never met criteria for Tourette's disorder or persistent (chronic) motor or vocal tic disorder, consider provisional tic disorder (full criteria are in DSM-5, p. 81).

vi. If a person experiences tics that do not meet criteria for a specific tic disorder because the movements or vocalizations are atypical in relation to age at onset or clinical presentation, consider other specified or unspecified tic disorder (see DSM-5, p. 85).

3. Attention-Deficit/Hyperactivity Disorder

a. Inclusion: Requires a pattern of behavior, with onset before age 12 years, that is present in multiple settings and gives rise to social, educational, or work performance difficulties. The symptoms must be persistently present for at least 6 months to a degree inconsistent with developmental level. The disorder is manifested by at least <u>six</u> of the following symptoms of inattention.

i. Overlooks details: *Over at least the last 6 months, have other people told you that you often overlook or miss details, or that you made careless mistakes in your work?*

ii. Task inattention: *Do you often have difficulty staying focused on a task or activity, such as reading a lengthy writing or listening to a lecture or conversation?*

iii. Appears not to listen: *Do other people tell you that when they speak to you, your mind often seems to be elsewhere or that it seems like you are not listening?*

iv. Fails to finish tasks: *Do you often struggle to finish schoolwork, chores, or work assignments because you lose focus or are easily sidetracked?*

v. Difficulty organizing tasks: *Do you often find it difficult to organize tasks or activities? Do you struggle with time management or fail to meet deadlines?*

vi. Avoids tasks requiring sustained mental activity: *Do you often avoid tasks that require sustained mental effort?*

vii. Often loses things necessary for tasks: *Do you often lose things that are essential for tasks or activities, such as school materials, books, tools, wallets, keys, paperwork, eyeglasses, or your phone?*

viii. Easily distracted: *Do you find that you are often easily distracted by things or thoughts unrelated to the activity or task you are supposed to be doing?*

ix. Often forgetful: *Do you find, or do other people find, that you are often forgetful in your daily activities?*

b. Inclusion: Alternatively, requires the presence of at least <u>six</u> of the following manifestations of hyperactivity and impulsivity over the same course.

    i. Fidgets: *Over the last 6 months, have you often found yourself fidgeting with your hands or feet? Do you find it hard to sit without squirming?*

    ii. Leaves seat: *When you are in a situation where you are expected to sit, do you often leave your seat?*

    iii. Runs or climbs: *Do you often find yourself running around or climbing in a situation where doing so is inappropriate?*

    iv. Unable to maintain quiet: *Do you often find yourself unable to play or engage in leisure activities quietly?*

    v. Hyperactivity: *Do you often feel as if you are, or do other people describe you as always being, on the go or acting as if you were "driven by a motor"? Do you find it uncomfortable to sit still for an extended time?*

    vi. Talks excessively: *Do you often talk excessively?*

    vii. Blurts answers: *Do you often struggle to wait your turn in a conversation? Do you often complete other people's sentences or blurt out an answer before a question has been completed?*

    viii. Struggles to take turns: *Do you often have difficulty waiting your turn or waiting in line?*

    ix. Interrupts or intrudes: *Do you often butt into other people's activities, conversations, or games? Do you often start using other people's things without permission?*

c. Exclusion: If the criteria are not met in two or more settings, or there is no evidence that the symptoms interfere with functioning, the symptoms occur only in the context of a psychotic disorder, or the symptoms are better explained by another mental disorder, do not make the diagnosis.

d. Modifiers

    i. Specifiers

- Combined presentation: If both inattention and hyperactivity-impulsivity criteria are met for the past 6 months
- Predominantly inattentive presentation: If inattention criteria are met but hyperactivity-impulsivity criteria have not been met for the past 6 months

- Predominantly hyperactive/impulsive presentation: If hyperactivity-impulsivity criteria are met and inattention criteria have not been met for the past 6 months

  ii. Specifiers
  - In partial remission
  iii. Severity
  - Mild: Few, if any, symptoms in excess of those required to make the diagnosis are present, and symptoms result in no more than minor impairments in social or occupational functioning.
  - Moderate: Symptoms or functional impairment between "mild" and "severe" is present.
  - Severe: Many symptoms in excess of those required to make the diagnosis, or several symptoms that are particularly severe, are present, or the symptoms result in marked impairment in social or occupational functioning.

e. Alternatives: If a person is experiencing subthreshold symptoms or you have not yet had sufficient opportunity to verify all criteria, consider other specified or unspecified attention-deficit/hyperactivity disorder (see DSM-5, pp. 65–66). The symptoms must be associated with impairment and do not occur exclusively during the course of schizophrenia or another psychotic disorder and are not better explained by another mental disorder.

Schizophrenia Spectrum and Other Psychotic Disorders

DSM-5 pp. 87–122

Screening questions: *Have you seen visions or other things that other people did not see? Have you heard noises, sounds, or voices that other people did not hear? Do you ever feel like people are following you or trying to hurt you in some way? Have you ever felt you had special powers, such as reading other people's minds? Have you ever been listening to the radio or TV and felt it was referring to you?*

If yes, ask: *Do these experiences influence your behavior or tell you to do things? Did these experiences ever cause you significant trouble with your friends or family, at work, or in another setting?*

- If yes, proceed to schizophrenia criteria.

1. Schizophrenia

   a. Inclusion: Requires at least 6 months of continuous signs of disturbance, which may include prodromal or residual symptoms. During at least 1 month of that period, at least <u>two</u> of the following symptoms are present, and at least <u>one</u> of the symptoms must be delusions, hallucinations, or disorganized speech.

      i. Delusions: *Is anyone working to harm or hurt you? When you read a book, watch television, or use a computer, do you ever find that there are messages intended just for you? Do you have special powers or abilities?*

      ii. Hallucinations: *When you are awake, do you ever hear a voice different from your own thoughts that other people cannot hear? When you are awake, do you ever see things that other people cannot see?*

      iii. Disorganized speech like frequent derailment or incoherence

      iv. Grossly disorganized or catatonic behavior

      v. Negative symptoms such as diminished emotional expression or avolition

   b. Exclusion: If the disturbance is attributable to the physiological effects of a substance (e.g., a drug of abuse, a medication) or another medical condition, do not make the diagnosis.

c. Exclusion: If a person has been diagnosed with autism spectrum disorder or a communication disorder of childhood onset, schizophrenia may be diagnosed only if prominent delusions or hallucinations are also present for at least 1 month.

d. Modifiers

  i. Specifiers

    • First episode, currently in acute episode
    • First episode, currently in partial remission
    • First episode, currently in full remission
    • Multiple episodes, currently in acute episode
    • Multiple episodes, currently in partial remission
    • Multiple episodes, currently in full remission
    • Continuous
    • Unspecified

  ii. Additional specifier

    • With catatonia: Use when at least <u>three</u> of the following are present: stupor, catalepsy, waxy flexibility, mutism, negativism, posturing, mannerisms, stereotypies, agitation, grimacing, echolalia, echopraxia.

  iii. Severity

    • Severity is rated by a quantitative assessment of the primary symptoms of psychosis, each of which may be rated for its current severity on a five-point scale (see Chapter 11, "Selected DSM-5 Assessment Measures," pp. 211–214).

e. Alternatives

  i. If a person has eccentric behaviors, perceptions, and thoughts and little capacity for close relationships, consider schizotypal personality disorder (full criteria are in DSM-5, pp. 655–656). If the disturbance occurs exclusively in the context of schizophrenia, a depressive or manic episode with psychotic features, or autism spectrum disorder, do not make the diagnosis.

  ii. If a person experiences only delusions, whether bizarre or nonbizarre, has never met full criteria for schizophrenia, and has functioning that is not markedly impaired beyond the ramifications of his delusion, consider delusional disorder (full criteria are in DSM-5, pp. 90–91). The criteria include multiple specifiers. This diagnosis should not be used if the delusions are due to the physiological effects of a substance or another medical condition. Do not use this diagnosis if the delusions are better explained by another mental disorder.

iii. If a person has experienced at least 1 day but less than 1 month of schizophrenia symptoms, consider brief psychotic disorder (full criteria are in DSM-5, p. 94). The person usually experiences an acute onset, exhibits fewer negative symptoms, and experiences less functional impairment, and always experiences an eventual return to his previous level of functioning.

iv. If a person has experienced at least 1 month but less than 6 months of schizophrenia symptoms, consider schizophreniform disorder (full criteria are in DSM-5, pp. 96–97). This diagnosis should not be used if the disturbance is due to the physiological effects of a substance or another medical condition.

v. If a person who meets criteria for schizophrenia also experiences major mood disturbances—either major depressive episodes or manic episodes—for at least half the time he has met criteria for schizophrenia, consider schizoaffective disorder (full criteria are in DSM-5, pp. 105–106). Over the person's lifetime, he must have experienced at least 2 weeks of delusions or hallucinations in the absence of a major mood episode.

vi. If a substance or medication directly causes a psychotic episode, consider substance/medication-induced psychotic disorder (full criteria are in DSM-5, pp. 110–111). The criteria include multiple specifiers for individual substances.

vii. If another medical condition directly causes the psychotic episode, consider psychotic disorder due to another medical condition (full criteria are in DSM-5, pp. 115–116). This diagnosis should not be used during an episode of delirium or when the psychotic episode is better explained by another mental disorder.

viii. If a person experiences psychotic symptoms that cause clinically significant distress or functional impairment without meeting full criteria for another psychotic disorder, consider unspecified schizophrenia spectrum and other psychotic disorder (see DSM-5, p. 122). If you wish to communicate the specific reason a person's symptoms do not meet the criteria, consider other specified schizophrenia spectrum and other psychotic disorder (see DSM-5, p. 122). Examples include persistent auditory hallucinations in the absence of any other feature and delusional symptoms in the partner of an individual with delusional disorder.

Bipolar and Related Disorders

DSM-5 pp. 123–154

Screening question: *Have there been times, lasting at least a few days, when you felt the opposite of depressed, when you were very cheerful or happy and this felt different from your normal self?*

If yes, ask: *During those times, did you feel this way all day or most of the day? Did those times ever last at least a week or result in your being hospitalized? Did these periods ever cause you significant trouble with your friends or family, at work, or in another setting?*

- If yes, proceed to bipolar I disorder criteria.
- If no, proceed to bipolar II disorder criteria.

1. Bipolar I Disorder

   a. Inclusion: Requires at least <u>three</u> of the following criteria during a manic episode.

      i. Inflated self-esteem or grandiosity: *During that period, did you feel especially confident, as though you could accomplish something extraordinary that you could not have done otherwise?*

      ii. Decreased need for sleep: *During that period, did you notice any change in how much sleep you needed to feel rested? Did you feel rested after less than 3 hours of sleep?*

      iii. More talkative than usual: *During that period, did anyone tell you that you talked more than usual or that it was hard to interrupt you?*

      iv. Flight of ideas: *During that period, were your thoughts racing? Did you have so many ideas you could not keep up with them?*

      v. Distractibility: *During that period, were you having more trouble than usual focusing? Did you find yourself easily distracted?*

      vi. Increased goal-directed activity: *During that period, how did you spend your time? Did you find yourself much more active than usual?*

      vii. Excessive involvement in activities that have a high potential for painful consequences: *During that period, did you engage in activities that were unusual for you? Did you spend money, use substances, or engage in sexual activities in a way that is unusual for you? Did any of these activities cause trouble for anyone?*

b. Exclusion: The occurrence of manic and major depressive episode(s) is not better explained by schizoaffective disorder, schizophrenia, schizophreniform disorder, delusional disorder, or other specified or unspecified schizophrenia spectrum and other psychotic disorder.

c. Exclusion: The episode is not due to the physiological effects of a substance or another medical condition. However, a manic episode that emerges during antidepressant treatment but persists beyond the physiological effect of the treatment meets criteria for the diagnosis.

d. Modifiers

   i. Current (or most recent) episode

      • Manic
      • Hypomanic
      • Depressed
      • Unspecified (use when the symptoms but not the duration of the criteria are met)

   ii. Specifiers

      • With anxious distress
      • With mixed features: Use if at least <u>three</u> of the symptoms of a major depressive episode are present simultaneously.
      • With rapid cycling
      • With melancholic features
      • With atypical features
      • With mood-congruent psychotic features
      • With mood-incongruent psychotic features
      • With catatonia
      • With peripartum onset
      • With seasonal pattern

   iii. Course and severity

      • Current or most recent episode manic, hypomanic, depressed, unspecified

         • Mild, moderate, severe
         • With psychotic features
         • In partial remission, in full remission
         • Unspecified

e. Alternatives

   i. If a substance directly causes the episode, including a substance prescribed to treat depression, consider substance/medication-induced bipolar and related disorder (full criteria are in DSM-5, pp. 142–143).

ii. If another medical condition causes the episode, consider bipolar and related disorder due to another medical condition (full criteria are in DSM-5, pp. 145–146).

2. Bipolar II Disorder

a. Inclusion: Requires at least <u>three</u> of the following criteria during a hypomanic episode lasting at least 4 days.

i. Inflated self-esteem or grandiosity: *During that period, did you feel especially confident, as though you could accomplish something extraordinary that you could not have done otherwise?*

ii. Decreased need for sleep: *During that period, did you notice any change in how much sleep you needed to feel rested? Did you feel rested after less than 3 hours of sleep?*

iii. More talkative than usual: *During that period, did anyone tell you that you talked more than usual or that it was hard to interrupt you?*

iv. Flight of ideas: *During that period, were your thoughts racing? Did you have so many ideas you could not keep up with them?*

v. Distractibility: *During that period, were you having more trouble than usual focusing? Did you find yourself easily distracted?*

vi. Increased goal-directed activity: *During that period, how did you spend your time? Did you find yourself much more active than usual?*

vii. Excessive involvement in activities that have a high potential for painful consequences: *During that period, did you engage in activities that were unusual for you? Did you spend money, use substances, or engage in sexual activities in a way that is unusual for you? Did any of these activities cause trouble for anyone?*

b. Exclusion: If there has ever been a manic episode or if the episode is attributable to the physiological effects of a substance/medication, the diagnosis is not given.

c. Exclusion: If the hypomanic episode is better explained by schizoaffective disorder, schizophrenia, schizophreniform disorder, delusional disorder, or other specified or unspecified schizophrenia spectrum and other psychotic disorder, the diagnosis is not given.

d. Modifiers

    i. Specify current or most recent episode

        • Hypomanic
        • Depressed

    ii. Specifiers

        • With anxious distress
        • With mixed features: Use if at least <u>three</u> of the symptoms of a major depressive episode are present simultaneously.
        • With rapid cycling
        • With mood-congruent psychotic features
        • With mood-incongruent psychotic features
        • With catatonia
        • With peripartum onset
        • With seasonal pattern
        • Unspecified

    iii. Course and severity

        • In partial remission
        • In full remission

        • Mild
        • Moderate
        • Severe

e. Alternatives

    i. If a person reports 2 or more years of multiple hypomanic and depressive symptoms that never rose to the level of a hypomanic or major depressive episode, consider cyclothymic disorder (full criteria are in DSM-5, pp. 139–140). During the same 2-year period (1 year in children and adolescents), the hypomanic and depressive periods have been present for at least half the time and the individual has not been without the symptoms for more than 2 months at a time. If the symptoms are due to the physiological effects of a substance or another medical condition, the diagnosis is not given.

ii. If a person experiences symptoms characteristic of bipolar disorder that cause clinically significant distress or functional impairment without meeting full criteria for a bipolar disorder, consider unspecified bipolar and related disorder (see DSM-5, p. 149). If you wish to communicate the specific reason a person's symptoms do not meet the criteria, consider other specified bipolar and related disorder (see DSM-5, p. 148). Examples include short-duration cyclothymia and hypomanic episode without prior major depressive episode.

Depressive Disorders

Screening questions: *Have you been feeling sad, blue, down, depressed, or irritable? Have you lost interest in, or do you get less pleasure from, the things you used to enjoy?*

    If yes, ask: *Did those times ever last at least 2 weeks? Did these periods ever cause you significant trouble with your friends or family, at work, or in another setting?*

- If yes, proceed to major depressive disorder criteria.
- If a child age 6 years or older says no, ask the irritability screening question, which appears after the alternatives for major depressive disorder below.

1. Major Depressive Disorder, Single and Recurrent Episodes

   a. Inclusion: Requires the presence of at least <u>five</u> of the following symptoms, which must include either depressed mood or lost of interest or pleasure (anhedonia), during the same 2-week episode.

      i. Depressed mood most of the day (already assessed)
      ii. Markedly diminished interest in activities or pleasures (already assessed)
      iii. Significant weight loss or gain: *During that period, did you notice any change in your appetite? Did you notice any change in your weight?*
      iv. Insomnia or hypersomnia: *During that period, how much and how well were you sleeping?*
      v. Psychomotor agitation or retardation: *During that period, did anyone tell you that you seemed to move faster or slower than usual?*
      vi. Fatigue or loss of energy: *During that period, what was your energy level like? Did anyone tell you that you seemed worn down or less energetic than usual?*
      vii. Feelings of worthlessness or excessive guilt: *During that period, did you feel tremendous regret or guilt about current or past events or relationships?*
      viii. Diminished concentration: *During that period, were you unable to make decisions or concentrate like you usually do?*
      ix. Recurrent thoughts of death or suicide: *During that period, did you think about death more than you*

usually do? Have you thought about hurting yourself or taking your own life?

b. Exclusion: If there has ever been a manic episode or a hypomanic episode, or the major depressive episode is attributable to the physiological effects of a substance or to another medical condition, the diagnosis is not given.

c. Exclusion: If the major depressive episode is better explained by schizoaffective disorder, schizophrenia, schizophreniform disorder, delusional disorder, or other specified or unspecified schizophrenia spectrum and other psychotic disorder, the diagnosis is not given.

d. Modifiers

   i. Specifiers

   • With anxious distress
   • With mixed features: Use if at least <u>three</u> of the symptoms of a major depressive episode are present simultaneously.
   • With melancholic features
   • With atypical features
   • With mood-congruent psychotic features
   • With mood-incongruent psychotic features
   • With catatonia
   • With peripartum onset
   • With seasonal pattern

   ii. Course and severity

   • Single episode
   • Recurrent episode

   • In partial remission
   • In full remission

   • Mild
   • Moderate
   • Severe
   • With psychotic features
   • Unspecified

e. Alternatives

   i. If a person reports experiencing depression or anhedonia for at least 2 years resulting in clinically significant distress or impairment, along with at least <u>two</u> of the symptoms of a major depressive episode, consider persistent depressive disorder (dysthymia) (full criteria are in DSM-5, pp. 168–169). If a person experiences 2 continuous months without depressive symptoms, do not give the diagnosis. If the person has ever had symptoms that met the criteria for a bipolar disorder or cyclothymic disorder, do not give the diagnosis. If the disturbance is better explained by a psychotic disorder or is due to the physiological effects of a substance or another medical condition, do not give the diagnosis.

ii. If a woman describes pronounced mood changes that begin in the week before her menses, decrease within a few days after the onset of menses, and abate in the week postmenses, consider premenstrual dysphoric disorder (full criteria are in DSM-5, pp. 171–172). The diagnostic criteria include at least <u>one</u> of the following: marked affective lability; marked irritability or interpersonal conflicts; marked depressed mood; and marked anxiety. At least <u>one</u> of the following symptoms must additionally be present (to reach a total of <u>five</u> symptoms when combined with the symptoms above): decreased interest in usual activities; subjective difficulty in concentration; lethargy, easy fatigability, or marked lack of energy; marked change in appetite; hypersomnia or insomnia; sense of being overwhelmed; and physical symptoms such as breast tenderness or swelling, joint/muscle pain, bloating, and weight gain.

iii. If a substance directly causes the episode, including a substance prescribed to treat depression, consider a substance/medication-induced depressive disorder (full criteria are in DSM-5, pp. 175–176).

iv. If another medical condition causes the episode, consider a depressive disorder due to another medical condition (full criteria are in DSM-5, pp. 180–181).

v. If a person experiences a depressive episode that causes clinically significant distress or functional impairment without meeting full criteria for a depressive disorder, consider unspecified depressive disorder (see DSM-5, p. 184). If you wish to communicate the specific reason a person's symptoms do not meet the criteria, consider other specified depressive disorder (see DSM-5, pp. 183–184). Examples include recurrent brief depression and depressive episode with insufficient symptoms.

Irritability screening question for children: *Do you ever lose your temper, yell, or act out?*
If yes, ask: *Do you lose your temper every day or every other day? Does your temper or yelling cause trouble at home or school?*

- If yes, proceed to disruptive mood dysregulation disorder criteria.
- If no, seek collateral information from caregivers or proceed to another diagnostic category.

2. Disruptive Mood Dysregulation Disorder

   a. Inclusion: Requires severe recurrent temper outbursts in response to common stressors, averaging at least three per week, for at least 1 year. The outbursts must occur in at least two distinct settings such as school or home, be severe in at least one setting, begin before age 10 years, and be characterized by the following three symptoms.

      i. Temper or behavioral outbursts: *When you get upset or lose your temper, what happens? Do you yell? Do you slap, punch, bite, or hit another person? Do you break or destroy things?*
      ii. Disproportionate reaction: *When you get upset or lose your temper, do you know what sets you off? What kinds of things bother you so much that you feel like yelling or hitting?*
      iii. Persistently irritable or angry mood between temper outbursts: *When you are not yelling or upset, how do you feel inside? Do you usually feel grouchy, angry, irritable, or sad?*

   b. Exclusion: These responses must be inconsistent with a child's developmental level.
   c. Exclusion: If the behaviors occur exclusively during an episode of major depressive disorder and are better explained by another mental disorder (e.g., autism spectrum disorder, posttraumatic stress disorder, sep-

aration anxiety disorder, persistent depressive disorder [dysthymia]), do not make the diagnosis.

d. Exclusion: If the symptoms are attributable to the
physiological effects of a substance or to another medical or neurological condition, do not make the diagnosis.

e. Exclusion: If a child is currently diagnosed with oppositional defiant disorder, intermittent explosive disorder, or bipolar disorder, do not make the diagnosis.

f. Alternative: If, during the last year, there was a period
lasting at least 1 day during which the child exhibited abnormally elevated mood and <u>three</u> criteria of a
manic episode, consider the possibility of a bipolar
disorder (see DSM-5, pp. 123–154).

Anxiety Disorders

DSM-5 pp. 189–233

Screening question: *During the past several months, have you frequently been worried about a number of things in your life? Is it hard for you to control or stop your worrying? A panic attack is a sudden rush of intense fear or anxiety that comes on from out of the blue for no apparent reason, or in situations where you did not expect it to occur. Have you experienced recurrent panic attacks? Do these experiences ever cause you significant trouble with your friends or family, at work, or in another setting?*

If yes, ask: *Can you identify specific objects, places, or social situations that make you feel very anxious or tearful?*

- If a specific phobia is elicited, proceed to specific phobia disorder criteria.
- If no, first proceed to panic disorder criteria. Then proceed to generalized anxiety disorder criteria.

1. Specific Phobia

   a. Inclusion: Requires that for at least 6 months, a person has experienced marked fear, anxiety, or avoidance as characterized by the following <u>three</u> symptoms.

      i. Specific fear: *Do you fear a specific object or situation such as flying, heights, animals, or something else so much that being exposed to it makes you feel immediately afraid or anxious? What is it?*

      ii. Fear or anxiety provoked by exposure: *When you encounter this, do you experience an immediate sense of fear or anxiety?* For children, ask, *When you encounter this, do you cry, experience tantrums, or hold on to a parent?*

      iii. Avoidance: *Do you find yourself taking steps to avoid this? What are they? When you have to encounter this, do you experience intense fear or anxiety?*

   b. Exclusion: The fear, anxiety, and avoidance are not restricted to objects or situations related to obsessions, reminders of traumatic events, separation from home or attachment figures, or social situations.

c. Modifiers

   i. Specifiers

      • Descriptive

         • Animal
         • Natural environment
         • Blood-injection injury
         • Situational
         • Other

d. Alternatives

   i. If a person reports developmentally inappropriate and excessive distress when separated from home or a major attachment figure, or expresses persistent worry that his major attachment figure will be harmed or has died, which results in reluctance or refusal to be separated from home or a major attachment figure, consider separation anxiety disorder (full criteria are in DSM-5, pp. 190–191). The onset of this disorder is before age 18. The minimum duration of symptoms necessary to meet the diagnostic criteria is 4 weeks for children and adolescents, but at least 6 months for adults.

   ii. If a person consistently fails to speak in specific social situations for at least 1 month, so that it interferes with educational or occupational achievement, consider selective mutism (full criteria are in DSM-5, p. 195). If the disturbance is due to a lack of knowledge of or comfort with the spoken language, do not give the diagnosis. If the disturbance is better explained by a communication disorder, autism spectrum disorder, or psychotic disorder, do not give the diagnosis.

   iii. If a person reports at least 6 months of marked and disproportionate fear or anxiety about situations such as public transportation, open spaces, being in enclosed spaces, standing in line or being in a crowd, or being outside the home alone, and if these fears cause him to actively avoid these situations, consider agoraphobia (full criteria are in DSM-5, pp. 217–218).

   iv. If a person reports at least 6 months of marked fear or anxiety about, or avoidance of, social situations in which he fears other people will observe or scrutinize him out of proportion to the actual threat posed by these social situations, and the fear, anxiety, or avoidance causes clinically significant distress or impairment, consider social anxiety disorder (social phobia) (full criteria are in DSM-5, pp. 202–203).

2. Panic Disorder

   a. Inclusion: Requires recurrent panic attacks, as characterized by at least <u>four</u> of the following symptoms:

      i. Palpitations, pounding heart, or accelerated heart rate: *When you experience these sudden surges of intense fear or discomfort, does your heart race or pound?*

      ii. Sweating: *During these events, do you find yourself sweating more than usual?*

      iii. Trembling or shaking: *During these events, do you shake or develop a tremor?*

      iv. Sensations of shortness of breath or smothering: *During these events, do you feel like you are being smothered or cannot catch your breath?*

      v. Feelings of choking: *During these events, do you feel as though you are choking, as if something is blocking your throat?*

      vi. Chest pain or discomfort: *During these events, do you feel intense pain or discomfort in your chest?*

      vii. Nausea or abdominal distress: *During these events, do you feel sick to your stomach or like you need to vomit?*

      viii. Feeling dizzy, unsteady, light-headed, or faint: *During these events, do you feel dizzy, light-headed, or like you may faint?*

      ix. Chills or heat sensations: *During these events, do you feel very cold and shiver, or do you feel intensely hot?*

      x. Paresthesias: *During these events, do you feel numbness or tingling?*

      xi. Derealization or depersonalization: *During these events, do you feel like people or places that are familiar to you are unreal, or that you are so detached from your body that it is like you are standing outside your body or watching yourself?*

      xii. Fear of losing control: *During these events, do you fear you may be losing control, or even "going crazy"?*

      xiii. Fear of dying: *During these events, do you fear you may be dying?*

b. Inclusion: At least <u>one</u> panic attack is followed by at least 1 month of at least one of the following symptoms:

    i. Persistent worry about consequences: *Are you persistently concerned or worried about additional panic attacks? Are you persistently concerned or worried that these attacks mean you are having a heart attack, losing control, or "going crazy"?*

    ii. Maladaptive change to avoid attacks: *Have you made significant maladaptive changes in your behavior, like avoiding unfamiliar situations or exercise, in order to avoid attacks?*

c. Exclusion: If the disturbance is better explained by another mental disorder or is attributable to the physiological effects of a substance/medication or another medical condition, do not make the diagnosis.

d. Alternatives

    i. If a person reports panic attacks as described above but neither experiences persistent worry about consequences nor makes significant maladaptive behavioral changes to avoid panic attacks, consider using the panic attack specifier (see DSM-5, p. 214). The panic attack specifier can be used with other anxiety disorders, as well as with depressive, traumatic, and substance use disorders.

3. Generalized Anxiety Disorder

a. Inclusion: Requires excessive anxiety and worry that is difficult to control, occurring more days than not for at least 6 months, about a number of events or activities, associated with at least <u>three</u> of the following symptoms.

    i. Restlessness: *When you think about events or activities that make you anxious or worried, do you often feel restless, on edge, or keyed up?*

    ii. Easily fatigued: *Do you find that you often tire or fatigue easily?*

    iii. Difficulty concentrating: *When you are anxious or worried, do you often found it hard to concentrate or find that your mind goes blank?*

    iv. Irritability: *When you are anxious or worried, do you often feel irritable or easily annoyed?*

    v. Muscle tension: *When you are anxious or worried, do you often experience muscle tightness or tension?*

vi. Sleep disturbance: *Do you find it difficult to fall asleep or stay asleep, or experience restless and unsatisfying sleep?*

b. Exclusion: If the anxiety and worry are better explained by another mental disorder or are attributable to the physiological effect of a substance/medication or another medical condition, do not make the diagnosis.

c. Alternatives

i. If a substance directly causes the episode, including a medication prescribed to treat a mental disorder, consider a substance/medication-induced anxiety disorder (full criteria are in DSM-5, pp. 226–227).

ii. If another medical condition directly causes the anxiety and worry, consider an anxiety disorder due to another medical condition (full criteria are in DSM-5, p. 230).

iii. If a person experiences symptoms characteristic of an anxiety disorder that cause clinically significant distress or functional impairment without meeting full criteria for another anxiety disorder, consider unspecified anxiety disorder (see DSM-5, p. 233). If you wish to communicate the specific reason a person's symptoms do not meet the criteria for a specific anxiety disorder, consider other specified anxiety disorder (see DSM-5, p. 233). Examples include *khyâl* (wind attacks), *ataque de nervios* (attack of nerves), and generalized anxiety not occurring more days than not.

Obsessive-Compulsive and Related Disorders

DSM-5 pp. 235–264

Screening questions: *Do you frequently experience unwanted images, thoughts, or urges? Are there any physical acts that you feel like you have to do in order to avoid or reduce the distress associated with these unwanted images, thoughts, or urges?*

   If yes, ask: *Do these experiences or behaviors ever cause you significant trouble with your friends or family, at work, or in another setting?*

- If yes, proceed to obsessive-compulsive disorder criteria.
- If no, proceed to body-focused repetitive behavior screening questions, which follow the obsessive-compulsive disorder section below.

1. Obsessive-Compulsive Disorder

   a. Inclusion: Requires the presence of obsessive thoughts, compulsive behaviors, or both, as manifested by the following symptoms.

      i. Obsessive thoughts (as defined by both questions): *When you experience these unwanted images, thoughts, or urges, do they make you really anxious or distressed? Do you have to work hard to ignore or suppress these kinds of thoughts?*

      ii. Compulsive behaviors (as defined by both questions): *Some people try to reverse intrusive ideas by repeatedly performing some kind of action such as hand washing or lock checking, or by a mental act such as counting, praying, or silently repeating words. Do you do something like that? Do you think that doing so will reduce your distress or prevent something you dread from occurring?*

   b. Inclusion: The obsessions or compulsions are time-consuming (e.g., take more than 1 hour per day) or cause clinically significant distress or impairment.

   c. Exclusions

      i. If the obsessions or compulsions are better explained by another mental disorder, do not make the diagnosis. If the obsessive-compulsive symptoms are due to the physiological effects of a substance or another medical condition, do not make the diagnosis.

ii. If a person reports that his intrusive images, thoughts, or urges are pleasurable, he does not meet the criteria for an obsessive-compulsive disorder. Instead, consider substance use disorders, personality disorders, and paraphilic disorders.

iii. If a person reports intrusive images, thoughts, or urges centered on more real-world concerns, consider an anxiety disorder.

d. Modifiers

i. Specifiers

- Insight

  - With good or fair insight: Use if a person recognizes that his beliefs are definitely or probably untrue.
  - With poor insight: Use if a person thinks his beliefs are probably true.
  - With absent insight/delusional beliefs: Use if a person is completely convinced his beliefs are true.

- Tic-related: Use if a person meets criteria for a current or lifetime chronic tic disorder.

e. Alternatives

i. If a person reports intrusive images, thoughts, or urges centered on his body image, consider body dysmorphic disorder (full criteria are in DSM-5, pp. 242–243). The criteria include preoccupation with perceived defects in physical appearance beyond concern about weight or body fat in a person with an eating disorder, repetitive behaviors or mental acts in response to concern about appearance, and clinically significant distress or impairments because of the preoccupation.

ii. If a person reports persistent difficulty in parting with possessions regardless of their value, consider hoarding disorder (full criteria are in DSM-5, p. 247). The criteria include strong urges to save items, distress associated with discarding items, and the accumulation of a large number of possessions that clutter the home or workplace to the extent that it can no longer be used for its intended function.

    iii. If a substance directly causes the condition, including a substance prescribed to treat depression, consider substance/medication-induced obsessive-compulsive and related disorder (full criteria are in DSM-5, pp. 257–258).

    iv. If another medical condition directly causes the episode, consider obsessive-compulsive and related disorder due to another medical condition (full criteria are in DSM-5, pp. 260–261).

    v. If a person experiences symptoms characteristic of an obsessive-compulsive and related disorder that cause clinically significant distress or functional impairment without meeting full criteria for another obsessive-compulsive and related disorder, consider unspecified obsessive-compulsive and related disorder (see DSM-5, p. 264). If you wish to communicate the specific reason a person's symptoms do not meet the criteria for a specific obsessive-compulsive and related disorder, consider other specified obsessive-compulsive and related disorder (see DSM-5, pp. 263–264). Examples include body-focused repetitive behavior disorder, obsessional jealousy, and *koro*.

2. Body-Focused Repetitive Behaviors

    a. Inclusion: DSM-5 includes two conditions, trichotillomania (hair-pulling disorder) and excoriation (skin-picking) disorder, with nearly identical criteria. Either diagnosis requires the presence of <u>all three</u> of the following symptoms.

        i. Behavior: *Do you frequently pull your hair or pick at your skin so much that it causes hair loss or skin lesions?*

        ii. Repeated attempts to change: *Have you repeatedly tried to decrease or stop this behavior?*

        iii. Impairment: *Does this behavior cause you to feel ashamed or out of control? Do you avoid work or social settings because of these behaviors?*

    b. Alternatives

        i. If the behavior is due to another medical condition, is better explained by another mental disorder, or is a result of substance use, you should not diagnose either trichotillomania or excoriation disorder.

Trauma- and Stressor-Related Disorders

DSM-5 pp. 265–290

Screening questions: *What is the worst thing that has ever happened to you? Have you ever experienced or witnessed an event in which you were seriously injured or your life was in danger, or you thought you were going to be seriously injured or endangered?*

If yes, ask: *Do you think about or reexperience these events? Does thinking about these experiences ever cause significant trouble with your friends or family, at work, or in another setting?*

- If yes, proceed to posttraumatic stress disorder criteria.
- If a child says no but his family or caregivers report disturbances in his primary attachments, proceed to reactive attachment disorder criteria.

1. Posttraumatic Stress Disorder

    a. Inclusion: Requires exposure to actual or threatened death, serious injury, or sexual violation. The exposure can be firsthand or witnessed. In addition, a person must experience at least <u>one</u> of the following intrusion symptoms for at least 1 month after the traumatic experience.

        i.   Memories: *After that experience, did you ever experience intrusive memories of the experience when you did not want to think about it?* For children, repetitive reenactment through play qualifies. *Do you repeatedly reenact that experience with your toys or dolls or when playing?*

        ii. Dreams: *Did you have recurrent, distressing dreams related to the experience?* For children, frightening dreams without recognizable content qualifies. *Do you frequently have very frightening dreams that you cannot recall or describe?*

        iii. Flashbacks: *After that experience, did you ever feel like it was happening to you again, like in a flashback where the event is happening again?* For children, this may be observed in their play.

        iv. Exposure distress: *When you are around people, places, and objects that remind you of that experience, do you feel intense or prolonged distress?*

        v.   Physiological reactions: *When you think about or are around people, places, and objects that remind you of*

that experience, do you have distressing physical responses?*

b. Inclusion: In addition, a person must experience at
    least <u>one</u> of the following avoidance symptoms for at
    least 1 month after the traumatic experience.

    i. Internal reminders: *Do you work hard to avoid
        thoughts, feelings, or physical sensations that bring up
        memories of this experience?*

    ii. External reminders: *Do you work hard to avoid peo-
        ple, places, and objects that bring up memories of this
        experience?*

c. Inclusion: In addition, a person must experience at
    least <u>two</u> of the following negative symptoms for at
    least 1 month.

    i.   Impaired memory: *Do you have trouble remembering
         important parts of the experience?*

    ii. Negative self-image: *Do you frequently think negative
         thoughts about yourself, other people, or the world?*

    iii. Blame: *Do you frequently blame yourself or others for
         your experience, even when you know that you or they
         were not responsible?*

    iv. Negative emotional state: *Do you stay down, angry,
         ashamed, or fearful most of the time?*

    v.   Decreased participation: *Are you much less inter-
         ested in activities in which you used to participate?*

    vi. Detachment: *Do you feel detached or estranged from
         the people in your life because of this experience?*

    vii. Inability to experience positive emotions: *Do you
         find that you cannot feel happy, loved, or satisfied? Do
         you feel numb, or like you cannot love?*

d. Inclusion: In addition, a person must experience at
    least <u>two</u> of the following arousal behaviors.

    i.   Irritable or aggressive: *Do you often act very grumpy
         or get aggressive?*

    ii. Reckless: *Do you often act reckless or self-destructive?*

    iii. Hypervigilance: *Are you always on edge or keyed up?*

    iv. Exaggerated startle: *Do you startle easily?*

    v.   Impaired concentration: *Do you often have trouble
         concentrating on a task or problem?*

    vi. Sleep disturbance: *Do you often have difficulty fall-
         ing asleep or staying asleep, or do you often wake up
         without feeling rested?*

e. Exclusion: The episode is not directly caused by a substance or by another medical condition.

f. Modifiers

  i. Subtypes

   • With dissociative symptoms, either depersonalization or derealization

   • Posttraumatic stress disorder for children 6 years and younger: Reserved for children under age 6 years who experienced trauma themselves, witnessed trauma, or learned of trauma experienced by a parent or other caregiver (full criteria are in DSM-5, pp. 272–274).

  ii. Specifiers

   • With delayed expression: Use if a person does not exhibit all the diagnostic criteria until at least 6 months after the traumatic experience.

g. Alternatives

  i. If the episode lasts less than 1 month and the experience occurred within the past month, and the person experiences at least <u>nine</u> of the posttraumatic symptoms described above, consider acute stress disorder (full criteria are in DSM-5, pp. 280–281).

  ii. If the episode began within 3 months of the experience and a person does not meet the symptomatic and behavioral criteria for posttraumatic stress disorder, consider an adjustment disorder (full criteria are in DSM-5, pp. 286–287). The criteria include marked distress disproportionate to an acute stressor, either traumatic or nontraumatic, and significant impairment in function.

  iii. If a person experiences symptoms characteristic of a trauma- and stressor-related disorder that cause clinically significant distress or functional impairment without meeting full criteria for one of the named disorders, consider unspecified trauma- and stressor-related disorder (see DSM-5, p. 290). If you wish to communicate the specific reason a person's symptoms do not meet the criteria for a specific trauma- and stressor-related disorder, consider other specified trauma- and stressor-related disorder (see DSM-5, p. 289). Examples include persistent complex bereavement disorder and adjustment-like disorder with delayed onset of symptoms that occur more than 3 months after the stressor.

2. Reactive Attachment Disorder

   a. Inclusion: Requires that a child experience extremes of insufficient care, before age 5 years, that result in <u>both</u> of the following behaviors.

      i. Rare or minimal comfort seeking: *When you are feeling really angry, upset, or sad, do you rarely seek comfort or consolation from other people?*

      ii. Rare or minimal response to comfort: *When you are feeling really angry, upset, or sad and somebody says or does something nice for you, do you find that you only feel a little better?*

   b. Inclusion: Requires the persistent experience of at least <u>two</u> of the following states.

      i. Relative lack of social and emotional responsiveness to others: *When you interact with other people, do you usually respond with very little feeling or emotion?*

      ii. Limited positive affect: *Do you usually find it hard to be excited, self-assured, and cheerful?*

      iii. Episodes of unexplained irritability, sadness, or fearfulness, which are evident during nonthreatening interactions with caregivers: *Do you often have episodes where you become irritable, sad, or afraid with an adult caregiver who does not pose a threat to you?*

   c. Inclusion: Requires the persistent experience of at least <u>one</u> of the following states.

      i. Social neglect or deprivation in the form of persistent lack of having basic emotional needs for comfort, stimulation, and affection met

      ii. Repeated changes of primary caregivers that limit opportunities to form stable attachments

      iii. Rearing in unusual settings that severely limit opportunities to form selective attachments

   d. Exclusions

      i. If a child does not have a developmental age of at least 9 months, do not make the diagnosis.

      ii. If a child meets criteria for autism spectrum disorder, do not make the diagnosis.

e. Modifiers
   i. Specifiers
      • Persistent: Use when the disorder is present for more than 12 months.
   ii. Severity: Specified severe when a child meets all symptoms of the disorder, with each symptom manifesting in relatively high levels
f. Alternative: If a young child who has experienced extremes of insufficient care exhibits profoundly disturbed externalizing behavior, consider disinhibited social engagement disorder (full criteria are in DSM-5, pp. 268–269). The criteria include at least <u>two</u> of the following symptoms: reduced reticence with unfamiliar adults, overly familiar verbal or physical behavior, diminished checking back with an adult caregiver after venturing away, and a willingness to go off with an unfamiliar adult with minimal or reduced hesitation.

Dissociative Disorders

DSM-5 pp. 291–307

Screening questions: *Everyone has trouble remembering things sometimes, but do you ever lose time, forget important details about yourself, or find evidence that you took part in events you cannot recall? Do you ever feel like people or places that are familiar to you are unreal, or that you are so detached from your body that it is like you are standing outside your body or watching yourself?*

    If yes, ask: *Did these experiences ever cause you significant trouble with your friends or family, at work, or in another setting?*

- If amnesia predominates, proceed to dissociative amnesia criteria.
- If depersonalization or derealization predominates, proceed to depersonalization/derealization disorder criteria.

1. Dissociative Amnesia

    a. Inclusion: Requires the presence of inability to recall important autobiographical information beyond ordinary forgetting, most often manifested by at least <u>one</u> of the following symptoms.

        i. Localized or selective amnesia: *Do you find yourself unable to recall a specific event or events in your life, especially events that were really stressful or even traumatic?*

        ii. Generalized amnesia: *Do you find yourself unable to recall important moments in your life history or details of your very identity?*

    b. Exclusions

        i. If the disturbance is better accounted for by dissociative identity disorder, posttraumatic stress disorder, acute stress disorder, somatic symptom disorder, or major or mild neurocognitive disorder, do not make the diagnosis.

        ii. If the disturbance is due to the physiological effects of a substance or a neurological or other medical condition, do not make the diagnosis.

    c. Modifiers

        i. Specifiers

            - With dissociative fugue: Use when a person engages in purposeful travel or bewildered wandering for which he has amnesia.

d. Alternatives

    i. If a person reports a disruption of identity, characterized by two or more distinct personality states or an experience of possession, that causes clinically significant distress and functional impairment, consider dissociative identity disorder (full criteria are in DSM-5, p. 292). The criteria include recurrent gaps in recall that are inconsistent with ordinary forgetting and dissociative experiences that are not a normal part of a broadly accepted cultural or religious practice and that are not attributable to the physiological effects of a substance or another medical condition.

2. Depersonalization/Derealization Disorder

  a. Inclusion: Requires at least <u>one</u> of the following manifestations.

    i. Depersonalization: *Do you frequently have experiences of unreality or detachment—like you are an outside observer of your mind, thoughts, feelings, sensations, body, or whole self?*

    ii. Derealization: *Do you frequently have experiences of unreality or detachment from your surroundings—like you often experience people or places as unreal, dreamlike, foggy, lifeless, or visually distorted?*

  b. Inclusion: Requires intact reality testing. *During these experiences, can you distinguish these experiences from actual events—what is occurring outside of you?*

  c. Exclusions

    i. If the disturbance is due to the physiological effects of a substance or a neurological or other medical condition, do not make the diagnosis.

    ii. If depersonalization or derealization occurs exclusively as symptoms of or during the course of another mental disorder, do not make the diagnosis.

  d. Alternatives

    i. If a person is experiencing a disorder whose most prominent symptoms are amnestic but does not meet the criteria for a specific disorder, consider other specified or unspecified dissociative disorder (see DSM-5, pp. 306–307). Examples include subthreshold dissociative disturbances in identity and memory, chronic and recurrent syndromes of mixed dissociative symptoms, identity disturbances in individuals subjected to prolonged periods of intense coercive persuasion, acute reactions to stressful situations, acute psychotic states intermixed with dissociative symptoms in a person who does not meet criteria for delirium or a psychotic disorder, and dissociative trance.

Somatic Symptom and Related Disorders

DSM-5 pp. 309–327

Screening questions: *Do you worry about your physical health more than most people? Do you get sick more often than most people?*

If yes, ask: *Do these experiences significantly affect your daily life?*

If yes, ask: *Which is worse for you, worrying about the symptoms you experience or worrying about your health and the possibility that you are sick?*

- If worry about symptoms predominates, proceed to somatic symptom disorder criteria.
- If worry about being ill or sick predominates, proceed to illness anxiety disorder criteria.

1. Somatic Symptom Disorder
   a. Inclusion: Requires at least <u>one</u> somatic symptom that is distressing. *Do you experience symptoms that cause you to feel anxious or distressed? Do these symptoms significantly disrupt your daily life?*
   b. Inclusion: Requires at least <u>one</u> of the following thoughts, feelings, or behaviors, typically for at least 6 months.
      i. Disproportionate thoughts: *How serious are your health concerns, and do you think about them often?*
      ii. Persistently high level of anxiety: *Do you persistently feel a high level of anxiety or worry about your health concerns?*
      iii. Excessive investment: *Do you find yourself investing a lot more time and energy into your health concerns than you would like to?*
   c. Modifiers
      i. Specifiers
         - With predominant pain
         - Persistent
      ii. Severity
         - Mild: One of the symptoms specified in (a) above
         - Moderate: Two or more of the symptoms specified in (a) above

- Severe: Two or more of the symptoms specified in (a) above plus multiple somatic complaints (or one very severe somatic symptom)

d. Alternatives

i. If a person is focused on the loss of bodily function rather than on the distress a particular symptom causes, consider conversion disorder (functional neurological symptom disorder) (full criteria are in DSM-5, pp. 318–319). The criteria for this disorder include symptoms or deficits affecting voluntary motor or sensory function, clinical evidence that these symptoms or deficits are inconsistent with a recognized medical or neurological disease, and significant impairment in social or occupational functioning.

ii. If a person has a documented medical condition other than a mental disorder, but behavioral or psychological factors adversely affect the course of his medical condition by delaying recovery, decrease adherence, significantly increase health risks, or influence the underlying pathophysiology, consider psychological factors affecting other medical conditions (full criteria are in DSM-5, p. 322).

iii. If a person falsifies physical or psychological signs or symptoms, or induces injury or disease to deceptively present himself to others as ill, impaired, or injured, consider factitious disorder imposed on self (full criteria are in DSM-5, p. 324). For the criteria to be met, the person needs to exhibit these behaviors even in the absence of obvious external rewards. The symptoms cannot be better accounted for by another mental disorder such as a psychotic disorder.

iv. If a person falsifies physical or psychological signs or symptoms, or induces injury or disease, to deceptively present someone else to others as ill, impaired, or injured, consider factitious disorder imposed on another (full criteria are in DSM-5, p. 325). The diagnosis is assigned to the perpetrator rather than the victim, and for the criteria to be met, the behavior needs to occur even in the absence of obvious external rewards, and not be better explained by another mental disorder such as a psychotic disorder.

2. Illness Anxiety Disorder

    a. Inclusion: Requires <u>all</u> of the following symptoms for at least 6 months and the <u>absence</u> of somatic symptoms.

        i. Preoccupation: *Do you find yourself unable to stop thinking about having or acquiring a serious illness?*

        ii. Anxiety: *Do you feel a high level of anxiety or worry about having or acquiring a serious illness?*

        iii. Associated behaviors: *Have these worries affected your behavior? Some people find themselves frequently checking their body for signs of illness, reading about illness all the time, or avoiding persons, places, or objects to ward off illness. Do you find yourself doing any of those things, or things like that?*

    b. Exclusion: If a person's symptoms are better explained by another mental disorder, do not make the diagnosis.

    c. Modifiers

        i. Subtypes

          • Care seeking
          • Care avoidant

        ii. Course

          • Transient

    d. Alternatives

        i. If a person endorses symptoms characteristic of a somatic symptom disorder that cause clinically significant distress or impairment without meeting the full criteria for a specific somatic symptom and related disorder, consider unspecified somatic symptom and related disorder (see DSM-5, p. 327). If you wish to communicate specific reasons that full criteria are not met, consider other specified somatic symptom and related disorder (see DSM-5, p. 327). Examples of other presentations in the other specified category include brief somatic symptom disorder, brief illness anxiety disorder, illness anxiety disorder without excessive health-related behaviors, and pseudocyesis.

Feeding and Eating Disorders

Screening questions: *What do you think of your appearance? Do you ever restrict or avoid particular foods so much that it negatively affects your health or weight?*

If yes, ask: *When you consider yourself, is the shape or weight of your body one of the most important things about you?*

- If yes, proceed to anorexia nervosa criteria.
- If no, proceed to avoidant/restrictive food intake disorder criteria.

1. Anorexia Nervosa

    a. Inclusion: Requires the presence of <u>all three</u> of the following features.

        i. Energy restriction leading to significantly low body weight adjusted for age, developmental trajectory, physical health, and sex: *Have you limited the food you eat to achieve a low body weight? What was the least you ever weighed? What do you weigh now?*

        ii. Fear of weight gain or behavior interfering with weight gain: *Have you ever experienced intense fear of gaining weight or becoming fat? Has there ever been a time when you were already at a low weight and still did things to interfere with gaining weight?*

        iii. Disturbance in self-perceived weight or shape: *How do you experience the weight and shape of your body? How do you think having a significantly low body weight will affect your physical health?*

    b. Modifiers

        i. Subtypes

            - Restricting type: Use when a person reports no recurrent episodes of bingeing or purging in the last 3 months.
            - Binge-eating/purging type: Use when a person reports recurrent episodes of bingeing or purging in the last 3 months.

        ii. Specifiers

            - In partial remission
            - In full remission

iii. Severity (based on body mass index [BMI])
- Mild: BMI $\geq$ 17 kg/m^2
- Moderate: BMI 16–16.99 kg/m^2
- Severe: BMI 15–15.99 kg/m^2
- Extreme: BMI < 15 kg/m^2

c. Alternatives

i. If a person reports recurrent binge eating, recurrent inappropriate compensatory behaviors to prevent weight gain (e.g., misuse of laxatives or other medications, self-induced vomiting, excessive exercise), and self-image unduly influenced by the shape or weight of his body, consider bulimia nervosa (full criteria are in DSM-5, p. 345). The diagnosis requires that binge eating and compensatory behaviors both occur, on average, at least once a week for 3 months. The diagnosis cannot be made if bingeing and compensating behaviors occur only during episodes of anorexia nervosa.

ii. If a person has recurrent episodes of binge eating characterized <u>both</u> by eating an amount of food that is definitely larger than most people would eat in a similar period of time under similar circumstances and by a sense of lack of control over eating during the episode, consider binge-eating disorder (full criteria are in DSM-5, p. 350). Binge-eating episodes are associated with at least <u>three</u> of the following: eating much more rapidly than normal, eating until feeling uncomfortably full, eating large amounts of food when not feeling physically hungry, eating alone because of feeling embarrassed by how much one is eating, and feeling disgusted with oneself, depressed, or very guilty after overeating. For the diagnosis to be made, a person must experience marked distress regarding the binge eating, and binge eating must occur, on average, at least once a week for 3 months. Finally, the binge eating cannot occur exclusively during the course of anorexia nervosa or bulimia nervosa.

2. Avoidant/Restrictive Food Intake Disorder

   a. Inclusion: Requires significant disturbance in eating or feeding as manifested by persistent failure to meet appropriate nutritional and/or energy needs associated with at least <u>one</u> of the following.

      i. Significant weight loss: *Do you avoid certain foods or restrict what you eat to the extent that it has seriously affected your weight? Have you experienced a significant weight loss as a result?* For children: *Do you avoid or restrict food to the extent that you have not grown at the expected rate?*

      ii. Significant nutritional deficiency: *Do you avoid or restrict food to the extent that it has negatively affected your health, as in experiencing a significant nutritional deficiency?*

      iii. Dependence on enteral feeding or oral supplements: *Have you avoided or restricted food to the extent that you depend on tube feedings or oral supplements to maintain nutrition?*

      iv. Marked interference with psychosocial functioning: *Has avoiding or restricting food impaired your ability to participate in your usual social activities or made it hard to form or sustain relationships? Can you eat with other people or participate in social activities when food is present?*

   b. Exclusion: If the eating disturbance is better explained by lack of available food or by an associated culturally sanctioned practice, or by eating practices related to a disturbance in body image, do not make the diagnosis.

   c. Exclusion: If the eating disturbance is due to another medical condition or is better explained by another mental disorder, do not make the diagnosis.

   d. Alternatives

      i. If a person persistently eats nonfood substances over a period of at least 1 month, consider pica (see DSM-5, pp. 329–330). The eating of nonnutritive, nonfood substances must be inappropriate to his developmental stage and must not be part of a culturally supported or socially normative practice.

      ii. If a person repeatedly regurgitates food over a period of at least 1 month, consider rumination disorder (full criteria are in DSM-5, p. 332). For this diagnosis, the regurgitation cannot occur as the result of an associated gastrointestinal or other medical condition, and the regurgitation cannot occur exclusively during the course of anorexia nervosa, bulimia nervosa, binge-eating disorder, or avoidant/restrictive food intake disorder.

iii. If a person has an atypical, mixed, or subthreshold disturbance in his eating and feeding, or if you lack sufficient information to make a more specific diagnosis, consider other specified or unspecified feeding and eating disorder (see DSM-5, pp. 353–354). DSM-5 also allows the use of this category for specific syndromes that are not formally included, such as purging disorder and night eating syndrome.

Elimination Disorders

DSM-5 pp. 355–360

Screening question: *Have you repeatedly passed urine or feces onto your clothing, your bed, the floor, or another inappropriate place?*

- If passing urine, proceed to enuresis criteria.
- If passing feces, proceed to encopresis criteria.

1. Enuresis

   a. Inclusion: In addition to the intentional or involuntary repeated voiding of urine into one's bed or clothes, requires the following frequency.

      i. Occurs at least twice a week for at least 3 consecutive weeks: *Has this occurred at least twice a week? Has it also occurred for 3 weeks in a row?*

   b. Exclusions

      i. If a person is younger than age 5 years, or the equivalent developmental age, do not make the diagnosis.

      ii. If the behavior is due to the physiological effects of a substance or another medical condition through a mechanism other than constipation, do not make the diagnosis.

   c. Modifiers

      i. Nocturnal only
      ii. Diurnal only
      iii. Nocturnal and diurnal

2. Encopresis

   a. Inclusion: In addition to the intentional or involuntary repeated voiding of feces into inappropriate places (e.g., clothing, floor), requires the following frequency.

      i. Occurs at least monthly for at least 3 consecutive months: *Has this occurred at least once a month? Has it also occurred for 3 months in a row?*

   b. Exclusions

      i. If a person is younger than 4 years, or the equivalent developmental age, do not make the diagnosis.

ii. If the behavior is attributable to the physiological effects of a substance or another medical condition through a mechanism other than constipation, do not make the diagnosis.

c. Modifiers

 i. With constipation and overflow incontinence
 ii. Without constipation and overflow incontinence

d. Alternatives

 i. If a person experiences symptoms characteristic of an elimination disorder that cause clinically significant distress or impairment without meeting the full criteria for an elimination disorder, consider unspecified elimination disorder (see DSM-5, p. 360). If you wish to communicate specific reasons that full criteria are not met, consider other specified elimination disorder (see DSM-5, p. 359).

Sleep-Wake Disorders

DSM-5 pp. 361–422

Screening questions: *Is your sleep often inadequate or of poor quality? Alternatively, do you often experience excessive sleepiness? Do you frequently experience an irrepressible need to sleep or experience sudden lapses into sleep? Have you, or has a sleeping partner, noticed any unusual behaviors while you sleep? Have you, or has a sleeping partner, noticed that you stop breathing or gasp for air while sleeping?*

- If dissatisfaction with sleep quantity or quality predominates, proceed to insomnia disorder criteria.
- If excessive sleep predominates, proceed to hypersomnolence disorder criteria.
- If an irrespressible need to sleep or sudden lapses into sleep predominate, proceed to narcolepsy criteria.
- If unusual sleep behaviors (parasomnias) predominate, proceed to restless legs syndrome criteria.
- If sleep breathing problems predominate, proceed to obstructive sleep apnea hypopnea criteria.

1. Insomnia Disorder

   a. Inclusion: Requires dissatisfaction with sleep quantity or quality, at least 3 nights per week, for at least 3 months, as manifested by at least <u>one</u> of the following symptoms.

      i. Difficulty initiating sleep: *Do you often have trouble getting to sleep?* For children: *Do you often have trouble getting to sleep without the help of a parent or someone else?*

      ii. Difficulty maintaining sleep: *After you get to sleep, do you frequently awaken when you do not want to wake up? Do you often have difficulty returning to sleep after these awakenings?* For children: *If you wake up when you wanted to be asleep, do you need the help of a parent or someone else to get back to sleep?*

      iii. Early-morning awakening: *Do you often wake up earlier than you intended and find yourself unable to return to sleep?*

   b. Exclusion: The sleep difficulty must occur despite adequate opportunity for sleep.

c. Exclusion: If the insomnia is better explained by or occurs exclusively during the course of another sleep-wake disorder, is attributable to the physiological effects of a substance, or is better explained by a coexisting mental disorder or medical condition, do not make the diagnosis.

d. Modifiers

   i. Specifiers

   - With non–sleep disorder mental comorbidity, including substance use disorders
   - With other medical comorbidity
   - With other sleep disorder

   ii. Course

   - Episodic
   - Recurrent
   - Persistent

e. Alternatives

   i. If a person experiences a persistent or recurrent pattern of sleep disruption leading to excessive sleepiness, insomnia, or both, and this disruption is primarily due to an alteration of the circadian system or to a misalignment between the endogenous circadian rhythm and the sleep-wake schedule required by the person's physical environment or social/professional schedule, consider a circadian rhythm sleep-wake disorder (full criteria, along with multiple subtypes, are in DSM-5, pp. 390–391). The sleep disturbance must cause clinical significant distress or functional impairment.

   ii. If substance use, intoxication, or withdrawal is etiologically related to insomnia, consider substance/medication-induced sleep disorder, insomnia type (full criteria, along with multiple subtypes, are in DSM-5, pp. 413–415). The disturbance cannot be better accounted for by delirium, a non-substance-induced sleep disorder, or the sleep symptoms usually associated with an intoxication or withdrawal syndrome. The disorder must cause significant distress or functional impairment.

   iii. If a person meets all criteria for an insomnia disorder but the duration has been less than 3 months, consider unspecified insomnia disorder (see DSM-5, pp. 420–421). The diagnosis is reserved for insomnia symptoms that produce significant distress or functional impairment. If you wish to communicate the reason a person's symptoms do not meet the full criteria for a specific sleep disorder, consider other specified insomnia disorder (see DSM-5, p. 420).

2. Hypersomnolence Disorder

   a. Inclusion: Requires excessive sleepiness at least three times per week for at least 3 months, despite a main sleep period lasting at least 7 hours, that causes significant distress or functional impairment. The hypersomnolence is manifested by at least <u>one</u> of the following symptoms.

      i. Recurrent periods of sleep: *Do you often have several periods of sleep within the same day?*
      ii. Prolonged nonrestorative sleep episode: *Do you often have a main sleep episode, lasting at least 9 hours, that is not refreshing or restorative?*
      iii. Sleep inertia: *Do you often have difficulty being fully awake? After an awakening, do you often feel groggy or notice that you have trouble engaging in tasks or activities that would otherwise be simple for you?*

   b. Exclusion: If the hypersomnia occurs exclusively during the course of another sleep disorder, is better accounted for by another sleep disorder, or is attributable to the physiological effects of a substance, do not make the diagnosis.

   c. Modifiers

      i. Specifiers

         • With mental disorder, including substance use disorders
         • With mental condition
         • With another sleep disorder

      ii. Course

         • Acute: Use when duration is less than 1 month.
         • Subacute: Use when duration is 1–3 months.
         • Persistent: Use when duration is greater than 3 months.

iii. Severity

- Mild: Difficulty maintaining daytime alertness 1–2 days/week
- Moderate: Difficulty maintaining daytime alertness 3–4 days/week
- Severe: Difficulty maintaining daytime alertness 5–7 days/week

d. Alternative: If substance use, intoxication, or withdrawal is etiologically related to daytime sleepiness, consider substance/medication-induced sleep disorder, daytime sleepiness type (full criteria, along with multiple subtypes, are in DSM-5, pp. 413–415). The disturbance cannot be better accounted for by delirium, a non-substance-induced sleep disorder, or the sleep symptoms usually associated with an intoxication or withdrawal syndrome. The disorder must cause significant distress or functional impairment.

3. Narcolepsy

a. Inclusion: Requires periods of an irrepressible need to sleep or lapsing into sleep, at least three times per week over the past 3 months, along with at least <u>one</u> of the following.

i. Episodes of cataplexy:

- For a person with long-standing narcolepsy: *At least a few times a month, do you find that after you laugh or joke, you suddenly lose muscle tone on both sides of your body but remain conscious?*
- For children or a person with ≤6 months of narcolepsy: *At least a few times a month, do you find that all of a sudden you grimace, open your mouth wide and thrust out your tongue, or lose muscle tone throughout your body?*

ii. Hypocretin deficiency: Measured using cerebrospinal fluid hypocretin-1 (CSF-1) immunoreactivity values.

iii. Nocturnal sleep polysomnography showing rapid eye movement (REM) sleep latency ≤15 minutes or a multiple sleep latency test showing mean sleep latency ≤8 minutes and ≥ sleep-onset REM periods.

b. Modifiers

  i. Subtypes

  - Narcolepsy without cataplexy but with hypo-cretin deficiency
  - Narcolepsy with cataplexy but without hypo-cretin deficiency
  - Autosomal dominant cerebellar ataxia, deaf-ness, and narcolepsy
  - Autosomal dominant narcolepsy, obesity, and type 2 diabetes
  - Narcolepsy secondary to another medical con-dition

  ii. Severity

  - Mild: Infrequent cataplexy (less than once per week), need for naps only once or twice per day, and less disturbed nocturnal sleep
  - Moderate: Cataplexy once daily or every few days, disturbed nocturnal sleep, and need for multiple naps daily
  - Severe: Drug-resistant cataplexy with multiple attacks daily, nearly constant sleepiness, and dis-turbed nocturnal sleep (i.e., movements, in-somnia, and vivid dreaming)

4. Obstructive Sleep Apnea Hypopnea

a. Inclusion: Requires repeated episodes of upper air-way obstruction during sleep. There must be polysom-nographic evidence of at least five obstructive apneas or hypopneas per hour of sleep, and <u>either</u> of the fol-lowing symptoms.

  i. Nocturnal breathing disturbances: *Do you often disturb your sleeping partner with snoring, snorting, gasping for air, or breathing pauses during sleep?*
  ii. Daytime sleepiness, fatigue, or nonrestorative sleep: *When you have an opportunity to get sleep, do you still wake up the next day feeling exhausted, sleepy, or fatigued?*

b. Inclusion: Alternatively, the diagnosis can be made by polysomnographic evidence of 15 or more obstructive apneas or hypopneas per hour of sleep regardless of accompanying symptoms.

c. Modifiers

   i. Severity

      • Mild: Use when a person's apnea hypopnea index is less than 15.
      • Moderate: Use when a person's apnea hypopnea index is between 15 and 30.
      • Severe: Use when a person's apnea hypopnea index is greater than 30.

d. Alternatives

   i. If a person demonstrates five or more central apneas per hour of sleep during polysomnographic examination, and this disturbance is not better accounted for by another current sleep disorder, consider central sleep apnea (full criteria are in DSM-5, pp. 383–384).

   ii. If a person demonstrates episodes of shallow breathing associated with arterial oxygen desaturation and/or elevated carbon dioxide levels during polysomnographic examination, and this disturbance is not better accounted for by another current sleep disorder, consider sleep-related hypoventilation (full criteria are in DSM-5, p. 387). This disorder is most commonly associated with medical or neurological disorders, obesity, medication use, or substance use disorders.

5. Restless Legs Syndrome

   a. Inclusion: Requires an urge to move the legs, usually accompanied by or in response to uncomfortable and unpleasant sensations in the legs, at least three times per week for at least 3 months, as manifested by all of the following symptoms.

      i. Urge to move legs: *While you are asleep, do you often experience uncomfortable or unpleasant sensations in the legs? Do you often experience an urge to move your legs?*

      ii. Relieved with movement: *Are these partially or completely relieved by moving your legs?*

      iii. Nocturnal worsening: *What times of day do you most experience the urge to move your legs? Is it worse in the evening or at night than during the day?*

b. Exclusions

   i. If these symptoms are attributable to a medical condition or to the physiological effects of a substance, or are better explained by another mental disorder or behavioral condition, do not make the diagnosis.

c. Alternatives

   i. If a person experiences recurrent episodes of incomplete awakening from sleep in which he experiences an abrupt and terrifying awakening (sleep terror) or he rises from bed and walks about (sleepwalking), usually during the first third of the major sleep episode, consider non–rapid eye movement sleep arousal disorders (full criteria are in DSM-5, p. 399). When experiencing an episode, the person experiences little to no dream imagery. The person experiences amnesia for the episode and is relatively unresponsive to efforts of other people.

   ii. If a person repeatedly experiences extremely dysphoric and well-remembered dreams and rapidly becomes alert and oriented upon awakening from these dysphoric dreams, consider nightmare disorder (full criteria are in DSM-5, p. 404). The dream disturbance, or the sleep disturbance produced by awakening from the nightmare, causes clinically significant distress or functional impairment. The dysphoric dreams do not occur exclusively during another mental disorder or are not a physiological effect of a substance/medication or another medical condition.

   iii. If a person repeatedly experiences episodes of arousal from sleep associated with vocalization and/or complex motor behaviors sufficient to result in injury to himself or his bed partner, consider rapid eye movement sleep behavior disorder (full criteria are in DSM-5, pp. 407–408). These behaviors arise during REM sleep and typically occur more than 90 minutes after sleep onset. Upon awakening, the person is fully awake, alert, and oriented. The diagnosis requires either polysomnographic evidence of REM sleep disturbance or evidence that the behaviors are injurious, potentially injurious, or disruptive.

iv. If substance or medication use, intoxication, or withdrawal is etiologically related to a parasomnia, consider substance/medication-induced sleep disorder, parasomnia type (full criteria are in DSM-5, pp. 413–415). The disturbance cannot be better accounted for by delirium, a non-substance-induced sleep disorder, or the sleep symptoms usually associated with an intoxication or withdrawal syndrome. The disorder must cause significant distress or functional impairment.

v. If a person has an atypical, mixed, or subthreshold disturbance in sleeping and waking, consider other specified or unspecified sleep-wake disorder (see DSM-5, pp. 421–422).

Sexual Dysfunctions

DSM-5 pp. 423–450

Screening question: *Have you been less interested in sex than usual or experienced difficulties in sexual performance?*

If yes, ask: *Have these experiences lasted at least 6 months and caused you significant distress or impairment?*

- If disinterest in sex predominates, proceed to female sexual interest/arousal disorder criteria for women or male hypoactive sexual desire disorder for men.
- If difficulties in sexual performance predominate, proceed to female orgasmic disorder for women or erectile disorder for men.

1. Erectile Disorder

    a. Inclusion: Requires the presence of at least <u>one</u> of the following symptoms on almost all or all occasions of sexual activity, for at least 6 months.

        i. Difficult to obtain: *During sexual activity, have you noticed a marked difficulty in obtaining an erection?*
        ii. Difficult to maintain: *Do you have a marked difficulty in maintaining an erection until the completion of sexual activity?*
        iii. Decrease in rigidity that interferes with activity: *Have you experienced a decrease in the rigidity of your erections severe enough that it interferes with sexual activity?*

    b. Exclusion: If a man has sexual dysfunction that is better accounted for by a nonsexual mental disorder, severe relationship distress, or another significant stressor, or is attributable to the effects of a substance/medication or another medical condition, do not make the diagnosis.

    c. Modifiers

        i. Subtypes

            - Generalized: Not limited to certain types of stimulation, situations, or partners
            - Situational: Only occurs with certain types of stimulation, situations, or partners

ii. Specifiers

- Lifelong: Disturbance has been present since the individual became sexually active.
- Acquired: Disturbance began after a period of relatively normal sexual function.

iii. Severity

- Mild: Evidence of mild distress over the symptoms
- Moderate: Evidence of moderate distress over the symptoms
- Severe: Evidence of severe or extreme distress over the symptoms

d. Alternatives

i. If a man reports that during almost all or all partnered sexual experiences over at least the last 6 months, he either did not ejaculate or experienced a marked delay in ejaculation, consider delayed ejaculation (full criteria are in DSM-5, p. 424). If the symptoms are better explained by a nonsexual mental disorder or severe relationship distress, do not give the diagnosis.

ii. If a man reports that he ejaculated within approximately 1 minute following vaginal penetration during almost all or all partnered experiences over at least the last 6 months, without wishing to do so, consider premature (early) ejaculation (full criteria are in DSM-5, pp. 443–444).

2. Female Orgasmic Disorder

a. Inclusion: Requires the presence of <u>one</u> of the following symptoms during all or almost all sexual experiences, for at least 6 months.

i. Delayed, absent, or infrequent orgasms: *Does it take you much longer than usual to achieve orgasm, or do you rarely or never experience an orgasm?*

ii. Reduced intensity of orgasms: *Have you noticed the intensity of your orgasms is markedly reduced?*

b. Exclusion: If a woman has sexual dysfunction that is better explained by a nonsexual mental disorder, severe relationship distress, or another significant stressor, or is attributable to the effects of a substance/

medication or another medical condition, do not make the diagnosis.

  c. Modifiers

    i. Subtypes

- Generalized: Not limited to certain types of stimulation, situations, or partners
- Situational: Only occurs with certain types of stimulation, situations, or partners

    ii. Specifiers

- Lifelong: Disturbance has been present since the individual became sexually active
- Acquired: Disturbance began after a period of relatively normal sexual function
- Never experienced an orgasm under any situation

    iii. Severity

- Mild: Evidence of mild distress over the symptoms
- Moderate: Evidence of moderate distress over the symptoms
- Severe: Evidence of severe or extreme distress over the symptoms

  d. Alternatives

    i. If a woman reports at least 6 months of marked difficulty having vaginal intercourse, marked vulvovaginal or pelvic pain during vaginal intercourse, marked fear or anxiety either about vulvovaginal or pelvic pain or vaginal penetration, or marked tensing or tightening of the pelvic floor muscles during attempted vaginal penetration, consider genito-pelvic pain/penetration disorder (full criteria are in DSM-5, p. 437).

3. Female Sexual Interest/Arousal Disorder

  a. Inclusion: Requires at least 6 months without, or with reduced, sexual interest or arousal as manifested by at least <u>three</u> of the following symptoms.

    i. Absent/reduced sexual interest: *Have you noticed that the intensity or frequency of your interest in sexual activity is absent or markedly reduced?*

    ii. Absent/reduced sexual thoughts: *Have you noticed that the intensity or frequency of your sexual thoughts or fantasies is absent or markedly reduced?*

    iii. No/reduced sexual initiation: *Have you noticed that the intensity or frequency with which you initiate sexual activity, or respond to a partner's initiation, is absent or markedly reduced?*

    iv. Absent/reduced sexual excitement/pleasure: *When you engage in sexual encounters, have you noticed that almost all of the time, your experience of sexual excitement or pleasure is absent or markedly reduced?*

    v. Absent/reduced sexual response: *Have you noticed that the intensity or frequency with which you experience sexual interest in response to erotic signals is absent or markedly reduced?*

    vi. Absent/reduced sexual sensations: *When you engage in sexual encounters, have you noticed that almost all of the time, the intensity or frequency with which you experience genital or nongenital sensation is absent or markedly reduced?*

b. Exclusion: If a woman has sexual dysfunction that is better accounted for by a nonsexual mental disorder, severe relationship distress, or another significant stressor, or is attributable to the effects of a substance/medication or another medical condition, do not make the diagnosis.

c. Modifiers

    i. Subtypes

- Generalized: Not limited to certain types of stimulation, situations, or partners
- Situational: Only occurs with certain types of stimulation, situations, or partners

- Lifelong: Disturbance has been present since the individual became sexually active
- Acquired: Disturbance began after a period of relatively normal sexual function

    ii. Severity

- Mild: Evidence of mild distress over the symptoms
- Moderate: Evidence of moderate distress over the symptoms

- Severe: Evidence of severe or extreme distress over the symptoms

d. Alternatives

   i. If a woman has a clinically significant disturbance in sexual function directly associated with the use or discontinuation of a substance or medication, consider a substance/medication-induced sexual dysfunction (full criteria are in DSM-5, pp. 446–447).

   ii. If a woman has a sexual dysfunction, but the symptoms do not meet the threshold for another sexual dysfunction diagnosis, the etiology is uncertain, or there is insufficient information to diagnose a current sexual dysfunction, consider unspecified sexual dysfunction (see DSM-5, p. 450). If you wish to communicate the specific reason a person's symptoms do not meet full criteria, consider other specified sexual dysfunction (see DSM-5, p. 450).

4. Male Hypoactive Sexual Desire Disorder

   a. Inclusion: Requires persistently or recurrently deficient (or absent) sexual thoughts or fantasies and desires for at least 6 months.

      i. Absent sexual thoughts: *Have you noticed that the intensity or frequency of your sexual thoughts, desires, or fantasies is absent or markedly reduced?*

   b. Exclusion: If a man has sexual dysfunction that is better accounted for by a nonsexual mental disorder, severe relationship distress, or another significant stressor, or is attributable to the effects of a substance/medication or another medical condition, do not make the diagnosis.

   c. Modifiers

      i. Subtypes

         - Generalized: Not limited to certain types of stimulation, situations, or partners
         - Situational: Only occurs with certain types of stimulation, situations, or partners

         - Lifelong: Disturbance has been present since the individual became sexually active
         - Acquired: Disturbance began after a period of relatively normal sexual function

ii. Severity

- Mild: Evidence of mild distress over the symptoms
- Moderate: Evidence of moderate distress over the symptoms
- Severe: Evidence of severe or extreme distress over the symptoms

d. Alternatives

i. If a man has a clinically significant disturbance in sexual function directly associated with the use or discontinuation of a substance or medication, consider a substance/medication-induced sexual dysfunction (full criteria are in DSM-5, pp. 446–447).

ii. If a man has a sexual dysfunction but the symptoms do not meet the threshold for another sexual dysfunction diagnosis, the etiology is uncertain, or there is insufficient information to diagnose a current sexual dysfunction, consider unspecified sexual dysfunction (see DSM-5, p. 450). If you wish to communicate the specific reason a person's symptoms do not meet full criteria, consider other specified sexual dysfunction (see DSM-5, p. 450).

Gender Dysphoria

DSM-5 pp. 451–459

Screening question: *Are you uncomfortable with your gender?*

If yes, ask: *Has this discomfort lasted at least 6 months and gotten to the point where you really feel like your given gender is incongruent with your gender identity? Does this discomfort cause significant trouble with your friends or family, at work, or in another setting?*

- If a child or his parent says yes, proceed to gender dysphoria in children.
- If an adolescent or adult says yes, proceed to gender dysphoria in adolescents and adults.

1. Gender Dysphoria in Children

    a. Inclusion: Requires at least <u>six</u> of the following manifestations (one of which must be a strong desire to be of the other gender), of at least 6 months' duration.

        i. Desire to be of other gender: *Have you experienced a strong desire to be of a gender other than your given gender? Do you insist that people treat you as a member of a gender other than your given gender?*

        ii. Cross-dressing: *Do you have a strong preference for clothes usually associated with a gender other than your given gender?*

        iii. Cross-gender fantasy: *When you play fantasy games, do you have a strong preference for cross-gender roles?*

        iv. Cross-gender play: *When you play, do you have a strong preference for toys or activities that most people associate with the other gender?*

        v. Cross-gender playmates: *Do you have a strong preference for friends of the other gender?*

        vi. Rejection of toys, games, and activities typically associated with other gender: *Do you strongly reject the toys, games, and activities typically associated with your given gender?*

        vii. Dislike of anatomy: *Do you have a strong dislike for your sexual anatomy?*

        viii. Desire to have other sex characteristics: *Have you experienced a strong desire for the primary or secondary sex characteristics that match your experience of gender?*

b. Specifiers

   • With a disorder of sex development

2. Gender Dysphoria in Adolescents and Adults

   a. Inclusion: Requires at least <u>two</u> of the following manifestations, of at least 6 months' duration.

      i.   Incongruence: *Have you experienced a profound sense that your primary or secondary sex characteristics do not match your gender identity?*

      ii. Desire to change: *Have you experienced a profound desire to change your primary or secondary sex characteristics because they do not match your gender identity?*

      iii. Desire to have sex characteristics of other gender: *Have you experienced a strong desire for the primary or secondary sex characteristics that match your experience of gender?*

      iv. Desire to be of other gender: *Have you experienced a strong desire to be of a gender other than your given gender?*

      v.   Desire to be treated as other gender: *Have you experienced a strong desire to be treated as a gender other than your given gender?*

      vi. Conviction that one has feelings of other gender: *Have you experienced a strong conviction that your typical feelings and reactions are those of the gender other than your given gender?*

   b. Modifiers

      i.   Specifiers

         • With a disorder of sex development

         • Posttransition: The individual has transitioned to full-time living in the desired gender (with or without legalization of gender change) and has undergone (or is preparing to have) at least one cross-sex medical procedure or treatment regimen

   c. Alternatives

      i.   If a person experiences symptoms characteristic of gender dysphoria that cause clinically significant distress or impairment without meeting the full criteria for gender dysphoria, consider unspecified gender dysphoria (see DSM-5, p. 459). If you wish to communicate the specific reason a person's symptoms do not meet full criteria, consider other specified gender dysphoria (see DSM-5, p. 459)

Disruptive, Impulse-Control, and Conduct Disorders

DSM-5 pp. 461–480

Screening questions: *Do you often have times when you become so upset that you make or even act upon verbal or physical threats to hurt other people, animals, or property? Have you ever been aggressive to people and animals, destroyed property, deceived other people, or stolen things?*

   If yes, ask: *Have these behaviors ever caused you significant trouble with your friends or family, at school or work, with the authorities, or in another setting?*

- If recurrent behavioral outbursts predominate, proceed to intermittent explosive disorder criteria.
- If recurrent rule breaking predominates, proceed to conduct disorder criteria.

1. Intermittent Explosive Disorder

   a. Inclusion: Requires recurrent behavioral outbursts in which the person does not control his aggressive impulses, as manifested by <u>either</u> of the following.

      i. Verbal or physical aggression: *Over the past 3 months, have you had impulsive outbursts in which you were verbally or physically aggressive toward other people, animals, or property? Have these outbursts occurred, on average, at least twice weekly?*
      ii. Three behavioral outbursts involving damage to or destruction of property and/or physical assault: *Over the last 12 months, have you lost control of your behavior three or more times and destroyed property or assaulted other people?*

   b. Inclusion: Also requires all <u>three</u> of the following.

      i. Magnitude of aggressiveness is disproportionate to any provocation or psychosocial stressor: *Looking back at these outbursts, can you identify any events or stressors associated with them? Was your response much more aggressive or extreme than these events or stressors?*
      ii. Recurrent outbursts are neither premeditated nor in pursuit of a tangible objective: *When you had these outbursts, did they happen when you were feeling angry*

or impulsive? Did the outburst occur without a clear goal like obtaining money or intimidating someone?

    iii. Outbursts cause marked personal distress, impair function, or are associated with financial or legal consequences: *How do these outbursts affect how you feel about yourself and how you get along with friends, family, and other people in your life? Have you ever suffered financial or legal consequences because of your outbursts?*

  c. Exclusions

    i. If the recurrent aggressive outbursts are fully explained by another mental disorder, or attributable to another medical condition or to the physiological effects of a substance/medication, do not make the diagnosis.

    ii. For children: If aggressive behavior occurs only in the context of an adjustment disorder, do not make the diagnosis. If chonological age, or equivalent developmental level, is less than 6 years, do not make the diagnosis.

2. Conduct Disorder

  a. Inclusion: Requires a repetitive and persistent pattern of behavior in which the basic rights of others or major age-appropriate societal norms or rules are violated, as manifested by the presence of at least <u>three</u> of the following in the past 12 months and at least <u>one</u> of the following in the past 6 months.

    i. Often bullies, threatens, or intimidates others: *Do you often bully, threaten, or intimidate other people?*

    ii. Often initiates physical fights: *Do you often start physical fights?*

    iii. Has used a weapon that can cause serious physical harm to others: *Have you used a weapon that could cause serious harm to someone else, such as a bat, brick, broken bottle, knife, or gun?*

    iv. Has been physically cruel to people: *Have you caused physical pain or suffering in other people?*

    v. Has been physically cruel to animals: *Have you caused physical pain or suffering in animals?*

    vi. Has stolen while confronting a victim: *Have you forcibly taken or stolen something from someone while the person was present?*

vii. Has forced someone into sexual activity: *Have you forced someone into sexual activity?*

viii. Has deliberately engaged in fire setting with the intention of causing serious damage: *Have you set fires in order to cause serious damage to a person, animal, or property?*

ix. Has deliberately destroyed others' property: *Have you deliberately destroyed someone else's belongings?*

x. Has broken into someone else's house, building, or car: *Have you broken into someone else's house, building, or car?*

xi. Often lies to obtain goods or favors or to avoid obligations: *Do you often lie to get out of work or to get things you want?*

xii. Has stolen items of nontrivial value without confronting a victim: *Have you taken or stolen something valuable from someone when the person was not present?*

xiii. Often stays out at night despite parental prohibitions, beginning before age 13: *Before the age of 13, did you have a curfew, a time after which you had to be at home, that you often violated by staying out later than you were supposed to?*

xiv. Has run away from home overnight at least twice while living in the parental or parental surrogate home (or once without returning for a lengthy period): *Have you ever run away from home? How many times? Did you ever run away from home and not return for a long time?*

xv. Is often truant from school, beginning before age 13: *Before the age of 13, did you often cut class or skip school?*

b. Exclusion: If a person is 18 years or older and meets the criteria for antisocial personality disorder, do not make the diagnosis.

c. Modifiers

i. Subtypes

- Childhood-onset type: Use when at least one criterion symptom begins before age 10 years.
- Adolescent-onset type: Use when no criterion symptoms are present before age 10 years.
- Unspecified onset: Use when the age at onset is unknown.

ii. Specifiers

- With limited prosocial emotions: Use for a person who persistently exhibits at least <u>two</u> of the following characteristics: lack of remorse or guilt, callous lack of empathy, lack of concern about performance, and shallow or deficient affect. To meet criteria, these characteristics must be displayed in multiple relationships and settings over at least 12 months. That is, these characteristics reflect a person's typical pattern of interpersonal and emotional functioning and not just occasional occurrences in some situations.

iii. Severity

- Mild: Few, if any, conduct problems beyond those required for diagnosis, and relatively minor harm to others
- Moderate
- Severe: Many conduct problems beyond those required for diagnosis, or considerable harm to others

d. Alternatives

i. If a person exhibits at least 6 months of a persistent pattern of angry and irritable mood along with defiant or vindictive behavior, consider oppositional defiant disorder (full criteria, along with specifiers, are in DSM-5, pp. 462–463). The pattern is manifested by at least <u>four</u> of the following: frequent loss of temper, being touchy or easily annoyed by others, being angry and resentful, arguing with authority figures, actively defying or refusing to comply with the requests or rules of authority figures, deliberately annoying people, blaming others for one's mistakes or misbehaviors, and at least two episodes of being spiteful or vindictive within the past 6 months. The behaviors must also cause clinically significant impairment and cannot occur exclusively during the course of a psychotic, substance use, depressive, or bipolar disorder, and the criteria for disruptive mood dysregulation disorder cannot be met. In addition, it is important to consider the persistence and frequency of these behaviors in relation to a person's developmental stage. For children younger than age 5, the behavior must occur on most days for at least 6 months. For children age 5 years or older, the behavior must occur at least once a week for at least 6 months.

ii. If a person reports deliberate and purposeful fire-setting on at least two occasions, consider pyromania (full criteria are in DSM-5, p. 476). The diagnosis requires tension or affective arousal before the fire setting, fascination with fire, and pleasure or relief when setting or witnessing fires. If the fire setting is done for monetary gain, to conceal criminal activity, out of anger, or in response to a hallucination, do not make the diagnosis. If the fire setting is better explained by intellectual disability, conduct disorder, mania, or antisocial personality disorder, do not make the diagnosis.

iii. If a person repeatedly fails to resist impulses to steal objects that are not needed for his personal use or their monetary value, consider kleptomania (full criteria are in DSM-5, p. 478). The diagnosis requires tension or affective arousal before the theft, and pleasure or relief at the time of the theft. If the stealing is done out of anger or vengeance, or in response to a hallucination, do not make the diagnosis. If the stealing is better explained by conduct disorder, mania, or antisocial personality disorder, do not make the diagnosis.

iv. If a person exhibits symptoms characteristic of a disruptive, impulse-control, and conduct disorder that cause clinically significant distress or impairment without meeting the full criteria for a diagnosis named above, consider unspecified disruptive, impulse-control, and conduct disorder (see DSM-5, p. 480). If you wish to communicate the specific reason a person does not meet the full criteria, consider other specified disruptive, impulse-control, and conduct disorder (see DSM-5, p. 479).

Substance-Related and Addictive Disorders

DSM-5 pp. 481–589

Screening questions: *How often do you drink alcohol? On the average day when you have at least one drink, how many drinks do you have? Have you had any problems as a result of drinking? When you stop drinking, do you go through withdrawal?*

Repeat for illicit and prescription drugs; begin by asking: *Have you ever experimented with drugs?*

After asking about drugs, ask: *Do you bet, wager, or gamble in a way that interferes with your life?*

If yes, ask: *Did these experiences ever cause you significant trouble with your friends or family, at work, or in another setting?*

- If a person reports problems with substance use, proceed to the substance use disorder criteria for the particular substance.
- If a person presents with substance intoxication, proceed to the substance intoxication criteria for the particular substance.
- If a person reports problems with substance withdrawal, proceed to the substance withdrawal criteria for the particular substance.
- If a person reports problems with gambling, proceed to gambling disorder criteria.

1. Alcohol Use Disorder

   a. Inclusion: Requires a problematic pattern of alcohol use leading to clinically significant impairment or distress as manifested by at least <u>two</u> of the following in a 12-month period.

      i. Drinking more alcohol over a longer period than intended: *When you drink, do you find that you drink more, or for a longer time, than you planned to?*

      ii. Persistent desire or unsuccessful effort to reduce alcohol use: *Do you want to cut back or stop drinking? Have you ever tried and failed to cut back or stop drinking?*

      iii. Great deal of time spent: *Do you spend a great deal of your time obtaining alcohol, drinking alcohol, or recovering from your alcohol use?*

iv. Cravings: *Do you experience strong desires or cravings to drink alcohol?*

v. Failure to fulfill major role obligations: *Have you repeatedly failed to fulfill major obligations at work, home, or school because of your alcohol use?*

vi. Continued use despite awareness of interpersonal or social problems: *Do you drink alcohol even though you suspect, or even know, that it creates or worsens interpersonal or social problems?*

vii. Giving up activities for alcohol: *Are there important social, occupational, or recreational activities that you have given up or reduced because of your alcohol use?*

viii. Use in hazardous situations: *Have you repeatedly used alcohol in situations in which it was physically hazardous, such as driving a car or operating a machine while intoxicated?*

ix. Continued use despite awareness of physical or psychological problems: *Do you drink alcohol even though you suspect, or even know, that it creates or worsens problems with your mind and body?*

x. Tolerance as manifested by <u>either</u> of the following.

- Markedly increased amounts: *Do you find that in order to get intoxicated or achieve the desired effect of drinking, you need to consume much more alcohol than you used to?*
- Markedly diminished effects: *If you drink the same amount of alcohol as you used to, do you find that it has a lot less effect on you than it used to?*

xi. Withdrawal as manifested by <u>either</u> of the following.

- Characteristic alcohol withdrawal syndrome: *When you stop drinking, do you undergo withdrawal?*
- The same or a closely related substance is taken to relieve or avoid withdrawal symptoms: *Have you ever drunk alcohol or taken another substance to prevent alcohol withdrawal?*

b. Modifiers

i. Specifiers

- In early remission
- In sustained remission
- In a controlled environment

ii. Severity

- Mild: Use when two or three criteria are present.
- Moderate: Use when four or five criteria are present.
- Severe: Use when six or more criteria are present.

c. Alternatives

  i. If a person received more than minimal exposure to alcohol at any time during gestation and experiences neurocognitive impairment, impaired self-regulation, and deficits in adaptive functioning, consider neurobehavioral disorder associated with prenatal alcohol exposure (an other specified neurodevelopmental disorder; see DSM-5, p. 86). The diagnosis requires onset of symptoms before age 18 years and clinically significant distress or functional impairment.

  ii. If a person experiences problems associated with the use of alcohol that are not classifiable as alcohol use disorder, alcohol intoxication, alcohol withdrawal, alcohol intoxication delirium, alcohol withdrawal delirium, alcohol-induced neurocognitive disorder, alcohol-induced psychotic disorder, alcohol-induced bipolar disorder, alcohol-induced depressive disorder, alcohol-induced anxiety disorder, alcohol-induced sexual dysfunction, or alcohol-induced sleep disorder, consider unspecified alcohol-related disorder (see DSM-5, p. 503).

2. Alcohol Intoxication

a. Inclusion: Requires at least <u>one</u> of the following signs or symptoms shortly after alcohol use.

  i. Slurred speech
  ii. Incoordination
  iii. Unsteady gait
  iv. Nystagmus
  v. Impairment in attention or memory
  vi. Stupor or coma

b. Inclusion: Requires clinically significant problematic behavioral or psychological changes. *Since you began this episode of drinking, have you observed any significant*

*changes in your behavior, mood, or judgment? Have you
done problematic things, or thought problematic thoughts,
that you would not have if you were sober?*

c. Exclusion: If the symptoms are due to another medical
condition or are better explained by another mental
disorder, including intoxication with another substance,
do not make the diagnosis.

3. Alcohol Withdrawal

a. Inclusion: Requires at least <u>two</u> of the following
symptoms, developing within several hours to a few
days of ceasing (or reducing) alcohol use that has been
heavy and prolonged.

   i.   Autonomic hyperactivity
   ii. Increased hand tremor
   iii. Insomnia: *Over the last couple of days, have you found it
        more difficult than usual to get to sleep and to stay asleep?*
   iv. Nausea or vomiting: *Over the last couple of days,
        have you felt sick to your stomach, felt nauseated, or
        even vomited?*
   v.   Transient visual, tactile, or auditory hallucinations
        or illusions: *Over the last couple of days, have you had
        any experiences where you worried that your mind was
        playing tricks on you, such as seeing, hearing, or feel-
        ing things that other people could not?*
   vi. Psychomotor agitation
   vii. Anxiety: *Over the last couple of days, have you felt
        more worried or anxious than usual?*
   viii. Generalized tonic-clonic seizures

b. Exclusion: If the symptoms are attributable to another
medical condition or better explained by another mental disorder, including intoxication with or withdrawal
from another substance, do not make the diagnosis.

c. Modifiers

   i.   Specifiers

        • With perceptual disturbances: Use when hallu-
           cinations occur with intact reality testing or
           when auditory, visual, or tactile illusions occur
           in the absence of delirium.

4. Caffeine Intoxication

a. Inclusion: Requires clinically significant problematic
behavioral or psychological changes shortly after caf-

feine ingestion, usually in excess of 250 mg (e.g., 2–3 cups of brewed coffee), as manifested by at least <u>five</u> of the following signs.

   i. Restlessness: *Over the last several hours, have you felt less able to remain at rest than usual?*

   ii. Nervousness: *Over the last several hours, have you felt more jittery or nervous than usual?*

   iii. Excitement: *Over the last several hours, have you felt more excited than usual?*

   iv. Insomnia: *Over the last several hours, if you tried to sleep, did you find it more difficult to get to sleep or stay asleep than usual?*

   v. Flushed face

   vi. Diuresis: *Over the last several hours, have you urinated more often or a greater amount than usual?*

   vii. Gastrointestinal disturbance: *Over the last several hours, have you experienced an upset stomach, nausea, vomiting, or diarrhea?*

   viii. Muscle twitching: *Over the last several hours, have you noticed your muscles twitching more than usual?*

   ix. Rambling flow of thought and speech: *Over the last several hours, have you or anyone else noticed that your thoughts or speech has been long-winded or even confused?*

   x. Tachycardia or cardiac arrhythmia

   xi. Periods of inexhaustibility: *Over the last several hours, have you felt like you had so much energy it could not be used up?*

   xii. Psychomotor agitation

b. Exclusion: If the symptoms are attributable to another medical condition or better explained by another mental disorder, including intoxication with another substance, do not make the diagnosis.

c. Alternative: If a person experiences problems associated with the use of caffeine that are not classifiable as caffeine intoxication, caffeine withdrawal, caffeine-induced anxiety disorder, or caffeine-induced sleep disorder, consider unspecified caffeine-related disorder (see DSM-5, p. 509).

5. Caffeine Withdrawal

a. Inclusion: Requires at least <u>three</u> of the following symptoms, developing within 24 hours of ceasing (or reducing) caffeine use that has been prolonged.

    i. Headache: *Over the last day, have you had any head-aches?*

    ii. Marked fatigue or drowsiness: *Over the last day, have you felt extremely tired or sleepy?*

    iii. Dysphoric or depressed mood or irritability: *Over the last day, have you felt more down, depressed, or even irritable than usual?*

    iv. Difficulty concentrating: *Over the last day, have you had difficulty staying focused on a task or activity?*

    v. Flu-like symptoms: *Over the last day, have you experienced flu-like symptoms, nausea, vomiting, or muscle pain or stiffness?*

  b. Exclusion: If the symptoms are attributable to another medical condition or are better explained by another mental disorder, including intoxication with or withdrawal from another substance, do not make the diagnosis.

6. Cannabis Use Disorder

  a. Inclusion: Requires a problematic pattern of cannabis use leading to clinically significant impairment or distress as manifested by at least <u>two</u> of the following in a 12-month period.

    i. Consuming more cannabis over a longer period than intended: *When you use cannabis, do you find that you use more, or for a longer time, than you planned to?*

    ii. Persistent desire or unsuccessful effort to reduce cannabis use: *Do you want to cut back or stop using cannabis? Have you ever tried and failed to cut back or stop?*

    iii. Great deal of time spent: *Do you spend a great deal of your time obtaining cannabis, using cannabis, or recovering from your cannabis use?*

    iv. Cravings: *Do you experience strong desires or cravings to use cannabis?*

    v. Failure to fulfill major role obligations: *Have you repeatedly failed to fulfill major obligations at work, home, or school because of your cannabis use?*

    vi. Continued use despite awareness of interpersonal or social problems: *Do you use cannabis even though you suspect, or even know, that it creates or worsens interpersonal or social problems?*

vii. Giving up activities for cannabis: *Are there important social, occupational, or recreational activities that you have given up or reduced because of your cannabis use?*

viii. Use in hazardous situations: *Have you repeatedly used cannabis in situations in which it was physically hazardous, such as driving a car or operating a machine while intoxicated?*

ix. Continued use despite awareness of physical or psychological problems: *Do you use cannabis even though you suspect, or even know, that it creates or worsens problems with your mind and body?*

x. Tolerance as manifested by <u>either</u> of the following.

- Markedly increased amounts: *Do you find that in order to get high or achieve the desired effect of using cannabis, you need to smoke or ingest much more cannabis than you used to?*
- Markedly diminished effects: *If you use the same amount of cannabis as you used to, do you find that it has a lot less effect on you than it used to?*

xi. Withdrawal as manifested by <u>either</u> of the following.

- Characteristic cannabis withdrawal syndrome: *When you stop using cannabis, do you undergo withdrawal?*
- The same or a related substance is taken to relieve or avoid withdrawal symptoms: *Have you used cannabis or another substance to prevent withdrawal?*

b. Modifiers

i. Specifiers

- In early remission
- In sustained remission
- In a controlled environment

ii. Severity

- Mild: Use when two or three criteria are present.
- Moderate: Use when four or five criteria are present.
- Severe: Use when six or more criteria are present.

c. Alternative: If a person experiences problems associated with the use of cannabis that are not classifiable as cannabis use disorder, cannabis intoxication, cannabis withdrawal, cannabis intoxication delirium, cannabis-induced psychotic disorder, cannabis-induced anxiety disorder, or cannabis-induced sleep disorder, consider unspecified cannabis-related disorder (see DSM-5, p. 519).

7. Cannabis Intoxication

   a. Inclusion: Requires at least <u>two</u> of the following signs or symptoms.

      i. Conjunctival injection
      ii. Increased appetite: *Over the last several hours, have you been much hungrier than usual?*
      iii. Dry mouth: *Over the last several hours, have you noticed that your mouth has been dry?*
      iv. Tachycardia

   b. Inclusion: Requires clinically significant problematic behavioral or psychological changes. *Since you began this episode of cannabis use, have you observed any significant changes in your mood, judgment, ability to interact with others, or sense of time? Have you done problematic things, or thought problematic thoughts, that you would not have without cannabis?*

   c. Exclusion: If the symptoms are due to another medical condition or better explained by another mental disorder, including intoxication with another substance, do not make the diagnosis.

   d. Modifiers

      i. With perceptual disturbances: Use when hallucinations occur with intact reality testing or when auditory, visual, or tactile illusions occur in the absence of delirium.

8. Cannabis Withdrawal

   a. Inclusion: Requires at least <u>three</u> of the following symptoms, developing within 1 week of ceasing (or reducing) cannabis use that has been heavy and prolonged.

      i. Irritability, anger, or aggression: *Over the last week or so, have you felt more irritable or angry, or like you were ready to confront or attack someone?*
      ii. Nervousness or anxiety: *Over the last week or so, have you felt more worried or anxious than usual?*
      iii. Sleep difficulty: *Over the last week or so, have you had any disturbing dreams or found it more difficult to get to sleep and to stay asleep than usual?*

iv. Decreased appetite or weight loss: *Over the last week or so, have you been less hungry or even lost weight?*

v. Restlessness: *Over the last week or so, have you felt less able to remain at rest than usual?*

vi. Depressed mood: *Over the last week or so, have you felt more down or depressed than usual?*

vii. Somatic symptoms causing significant discomfort: *Over the last week or so, have you felt any unusual physical discomfort, such as stomach pain, tremors, sweating, fever, chills, or headaches?*

b. Exclusion: If the symptoms are attributable to another medical condition or better explained by another mental disorder, including intoxication with or withdrawal from another substance, do not make the diagnosis.

9. Phencyclidine or Other Hallucinogen Use Disorder

a. Inclusion: Requires a problematic pattern of phencyclidine or other hallucinogen use leading to clinically significant impairment or distress as manifested by at least <u>two</u> of the following in a 12-month period.

i. Using more phencyclidine or other hallucinogens over a longer period than intended: *When you use hallucinogens, do you find that you use more, or for a longer time, than you planned to?*

ii. Persistent desire or unsuccessful effort to reduce hallucinogen use: *Do you want to cut back or stop using hallucinogens? Have you ever tried and failed to cut back or stop using hallucinogens?*

iii. Great deal of time spent: *Do you spend a great deal of your time obtaining hallucinogens, using hallucinogens, or recovering from your hallucinogen use?*

iv. Cravings: *Do you experience strong desires or cravings to use hallucinogens?*

v. Failure to fulfill major role obligations: *Have you repeatedly failed to fulfill major obligations at work, home, or school because of your hallucinogen use?*

vi. Continued use despite awareness of interpersonal or social problems: *Do you use hallucinogens even though you suspect, or even know, that your use creates or worsens interpersonal or social problems?*

vii. Giving up activities for hallucinogens: *Are there important social, occupational, or recreational activi-*

ties that you have given up or reduced because of your hallucinogen use?

viii. Use in hazardous situations: *Have you repeatedly used hallucinogens in situations in which it was physically hazardous, such as driving a car or operating a machine while impaired by a hallucinogen?*

ix. Continued use despite awareness of physical or psychological problems: *Do you use hallucinogens even though you suspect, or even know, that they create or worsen problems with your mind and body?*

x. Tolerance as manifested by <u>either</u> of the following.

- Markedly increased amounts: *Do you find that in order to achieve the desired effect of hallucinogens, you need to consume much more than you used to?*
- Markedly diminished effects: *If you use the same amount of a hallucinogen as you used to, do you find that it has a lot less effect on you than it used to?*

b. Modifiers

i. Specifiers

- In early remission
- In sustained remission
- In a controlled environment

ii. Severity

- Mild: Use when two or three criteria are present.
- Moderate: Use when four or five criteria are present.
- Severe: Use when six or more criteria are present.

c. Alternatives:

i. If a person reports reexperiencing perceptual symptoms he first experienced while impaired by a hallucinogen after ceasing use, consider hallucinogen persisting perception disorder (full criteria are in DSM-5, p. 531). The symptoms must cause clinically significant distress or impairment.

ii. If a person experiences problems associated with the use of phencyclidine or other hallucinogens that are not classifiable as phencyclidine or other halluci-

nogen use disorder, phencyclidine or other hallucinogen intoxication, hallucinogen persisting perception disorder, phencyclidine or other hallucinogen
intoxication delirium, phencyclidine- or other hallucinogen-induced psychotic disorder, phencycli-
dine- or other hallucinogen–induced bipolar disorder, phencyclidine- or other hallucinogen-induced
depressive disorder, or phencyclidine- or other hal-
lucinogen- anxiety disorder, consider unspecified
phencyclidine-related disorder or unspecified hal-
lucinogen-related disorder (see DSM-5, p. 533).

10. Phencyclidine or Other Hallucinogen Intoxication

   a. Inclusion: Requires at least <u>two</u> of the following signs
      shortly after hallucinogen use.

   Phencyclidine
      i. Vertical or horizontal nystagmus
      ii. Hypertension or tachycardia
      iii. Numbness or diminished responsiveness to pain
      iv. Ataxia
      v. Dysarthria
      vi. Muscle rigidity
      vii. Seizures or coma
      viii. Hyperacusis

   Other hallucinogens
      i. Pupillary dilation
      ii. Tachycardia
      iii. Sweating: *Since taking the hallucinogen, have you no-
           ticed any change in how much you sweat?*
      iv. Palpitations: *Since taking the hallucinogen, has your
          heartbeat been more rapid, strong, or irregular than
          usual?*
      v. Blurring of vision: *Since taking the hallucinogen, has
         your vision been blurred?*
      vi. Tremors
      vii. Incoordination: *Since taking the hallucinogen, have
           you found it hard to coordinate your movements as you
           walk or otherwise move?*

   b. Inclusion: Requires clinically significant problematic
      behavioral or psychological changes. *Since you began
      this episode of hallucinogen use, have you observed any sig-
      nificant changes in your thoughts or behaviors? Have you*

done problematic things, or thought problematic thoughts, that you would not have without hallucinogens?

c. Exclusion: If the symptoms are attributable to another medical condition or better explained by another mental disorder, including intoxication with another substance, do not make the diagnosis.

11. Inhalant Use Disorder

   a. Inclusion: Requires a problematic pattern of inhalant use leading to clinically significant impairment or distress as manifested by at least <u>two</u> of the following in a 12-month period.

      i. Using more inhalants over a longer period than intended: *When you inhale, do you find that you use more inhalant, or for a longer time, than you planned to?*

      ii. Persistent desire or unsuccessful effort to reduce inhalant use: *Do you want to cut back or stop inhaling? Have you ever tried and failed to cut back or stop inhaling?*

      iii. Great deal of time spent: *Do you spend a great deal of your time obtaining inhalants, using inhalants, or recovering from your inhalant use?*

      iv. Cravings: *Do you experience strong desires or cravings to use inhalants?*

      v. Failure to fulfill major role obligations: *Have you repeatedly failed to fulfill major obligations at work, home, or school because of your inhalant use?*

      vi. Continued use despite awareness of interpersonal or social problems: *Do you use inhalants even though you suspect, or even know, that your use creates or worsens interpersonal or social problems?*

      vii. Giving up activities for inhalants: *Are there important social, occupational, or recreational activities that you have given up or reduced because of your inhalant use?*

      viii. Use in hazardous situations: *Have you repeatedly used inhalants in situations in which it was physically hazardous, such as driving a car or operating a machine while high?*

      ix. Continued use despite awareness of physical or psychological problems: *Do you use inhalants even though you suspect, or even know, that it creates or worsens problems with your mind and body?*

x. Tolerance as manifested by <u>either</u> of the following.

- Markedly increased amounts: *Do you find that in order to get high or achieve the desired effect of using inhalants, you need to use much more than you used to?*
- Markedly diminished effects: *If you inhale the same amount of an inhalant as you used to, do you find that it has a lot less effect on you than it used to?*

b. Modifiers

  i. Specifiers

  - In early remission
  - In sustained remission
  - In a controlled environment

  ii. Severity

  - Mild: Use when two or three criteria are present.
  - Moderate: Use when four or five criteria are present.
  - Severe: Use when six or more criteria are present.

c. Alternative: If a person experiences problems associated with the use of an inhalant that are not classifiable as inhalant use disorder, inhalant intoxication, inhalant intoxication delirium, inhalant-induced major or mild neurocognitive disorder, inhalant-induced psychotic disorder, inhalant-induced depressive disorder, or inhalant-induced anxiety disorder, consider unspecified inhalant-related disorder (see DSM-5, p. 540).

12. Inhalant Intoxication

a. Inclusion: Requires at least <u>two</u> of the following signs after intended or unintended short-term, high-dose inhalant exposure.

  i. Dizziness: *Since using the inhalant, have you felt like you were reeling or about to fall?*
  ii. Nystagmus
  iii. Incoordination: *Since using the inhalant, have you found it hard to coordinate your movements as you walk or otherwise move?*
  iv. Slurred speech
  v. Unsteady gait
  vi. Lethargy: *Since using the inhalant, have you felt very sleepy or had a marked lack of energy?*

vii. Depressed reflexes
viii. Psychomotor retardation
ix. Tremor
x. Generalized muscle weakness
xi. Blurred vision or diplopia: *Since using the inhalant, has your vision been blurred or have you been seeing double?*
xii. Stupor or coma
xiii. Euphoria: *Since using the inhalant, have you felt mentally or physically elated or intensely excited or happy?*

b. Inclusion: Requires clinically significant problematic behavioral or psychological changes. *Since you began this episode of inhalant use, have you observed any significant changes in your thoughts or behaviors? Have you done problematic things, or thought problematic thoughts, that you would not have without the inhalant?*

c. Exclusion: If the symptoms are attributable to another medical condition or better explained by another mental disorder, including intoxication with another substance, do not make the diagnosis.

13. Opioid Use Disorder

a. Inclusion: Requires a problematic pattern of opioid use leading to clinically significant impairment or distress as manifested by at least <u>two</u> of the following in a 12-month period.

i. Using more opioids over a longer period than intended: *When you use opioids, do you find that you use more, or for a longer time, than you planned to?*

ii. Persistent desire or unsuccessful effort to reduce opioid use: *Do you want to cut back or stop using opioids? Have you ever tried and failed to cut back or stop your opioid use?*

iii. Great deal of time spent: *Do you spend a great deal of your time obtaining opioids, using opioids, or recovering from your opioid use?*

iv. Cravings: *Do you experience strong desires or cravings to use opioids?*

v. Failure to fulfill major role obligations: *Have you repeatedly failed to fulfill major obligations at work, home, or school because of your opioid use?*

vi. Continued use despite awareness of interpersonal or social problems: *Do you continue to use opioids even though you suspect, or even know, that your use creates or worsens interpersonal or social problems?*

vii. Giving up activities for opioids: *Are there important social, occupational, or recreational activities that you have given up or reduced because of your opioid use?*

viii. Use in hazardous situations: *Have you repeatedly used opioids in situations in which it was physically hazardous, such as driving a car or operating a machine while intoxicated?*

ix. Continued use despite awareness of physical or psychological problems: *Do you use opioids even though you suspect, or even know, that it creates or worsens problems with your mind and body?*

x. Tolerance as manifested by <u>either</u> of the following.

- Markedly increased amounts: *Do you find that in order to get high or achieve the desired effect of using opioids, you need to consume much more than you used to?*

- Markedly diminished effects (excluding opioid medications taken under medical supervision): *If you use the same amount of an opioid as you used to, do you find that it has a lot less effect on you than it used to?*

xi. Withdrawal as manifested by <u>either</u> of the following.

- Characteristic opioid withdrawal syndrome: *When you stop using opioids, do you undergo withdrawal?*

- The same or a closely related substance is taken to relieve or avoid withdrawal symptoms: *Have you ever taken opioids or another substance to prevent opioid withdrawal?*

b. Modifiers

i. Specifiers

- In early remission
- In sustained remission
- On maintenance therapy
- In a controlled environment

ii. Severity

- Mild: Use when two or three criteria are present.
- Moderate: Use when four or five criteria are present.
- Severe: Use when six or more criteria are present.

The DSM-5 Diagnostic Interview   **143**

c. Alternative: If a person experiences problems associated with the use of opioids that are not classifiable as opioid use disorder, opioid intoxication, opioid withdrawal, opioid intoxication delirium, opioid withdrawal delirium, opioid-induced psychotic disorder, opioid-induced bipolar disorder, opioid-induced depressive disorder, opioid-induced anxiety disorder, opioid-induced sexual dysfunction, or opioid-induced sleep disorder, consider unspecified opioid-related disorder (see DSM-5, p. 550).

14. Opioid Intoxication

   a. Inclusion: Requires pupillary constriction shortly after opioid use and at least <u>one</u> of the following signs.

      i. Drowsiness or coma
      ii. Slurred speech
      iii. Impairment in attention or memory

   b. Inclusion: Requires clinically significant problematic behavioral or psychological changes. *Since you began this episode of opioid use, have you observed any significant changes in your thoughts or behaviors? Have you done problematic things, or thought problematic thoughts, that you would not have without the opioid?*

   c. Exclusion: If the symptoms are attributable to another medical condition or better explained by another mental disorder, including intoxication with another substance, do not make the diagnosis.

   d. Modifiers

      i. With perceptual disturbances: Use when hallucinations occur with intact reality testing or when auditory, visual, or tactile illusions occur in the absence of delirium.

15. Opioid Withdrawal

   a. Inclusion: Requires at least <u>three</u> of the following symptoms, developing within minutes to several days of ceasing (or reducing) opioid use that has been heavy and prolonged OR following the administration of an opioid antagonist after a period of opioid use.

      i. Dysphoric mood: *Over the last couple of days, have you been feeling more down or depressed than usual?*
      ii. Nausea or vomiting: *Over the last couple of days, have you felt sick to your stomach, felt nauseated, or even vomited?*

iii. Muscle aches: *Over the last couple of days, have you experienced muscle aches or pains?*

iv. Lacrimation or rhinorrhea: *Over the last couple of days, have you noticed that you have been shedding tears when you did not feel like crying? Have you noticed that your nose has been running, or discharging clear fluid, more than usual?*

v. Pupillary dilation, piloerection, or sweating

vi. Diarrhea: *Over the last couple of days, have you experienced more frequent or more liquid stools than usual?*

vii. Yawning: *Over the last couple of days, have you been yawning much more than usual?*

viii. Fever

ix. Insomnia: *Over the last couple of days, have you found it more difficult than usual to get to sleep and to stay asleep?*

b. Exclusion: If the symptoms are attributable to another medical condition or better explained by another mental disorder, including intoxication with or withdrawal from another substance, do not make the diagnosis.

16. Sedative, Hypnotic, or Anxiolytic Use Disorder

a. Inclusion: Requires a problematic pattern of sedative, hypnotic, or anxiolytic use leading to clinically significant impairment or distress as manifested by at least <u>two</u> of the following in a 12-month period.

i. Using more sedatives, hypnotics, or anxiolytics over a longer period than intended: *When you use sedatives, hypnotics, or anxiolytics, do you find that you use more, and for a longer time, than you planned to?*

ii. Persistent desire or unsuccessful effort to reduce sedative, hypnotic, or anxiolytic use: *Do you want to cut back or stop using sedatives, hypnotics, or anxiolytics? Have you ever tried and failed to cut back or stop using sedatives, hypnotics, or anxiolytics?*

iii. Great deal of time spent: *Do you spend a great deal of your time obtaining and using sedatives, hypnotics, or anxiolytics or recovering from your sedative, hypnotic, or anxiolytic use?*

iv. Cravings: *Do you experience strong desires or cravings to use sedatives, hypnotics, or anxiolytics?*

v. Failure to fulfill major role obligations: *Have you repeatedly failed to fulfill major obligations at work, home, or school because of your sedative, hypnotic, or anxiolytic use?*

vi. Continued use despite awareness of interpersonal or social problems: *Do you use a sedative, hypnotic, or anxiolytic even though you suspect, or even know, that it creates or worsens interpersonal or social problems?*

vii. Giving up activities for sedatives, hypnotics, or anxiolytics: *Are there important social, occupational, or recreational activities that you have given up or reduced because of your sedative, hypnotic, or anxiolytic use?*

viii. Use in hazardous situations: *Have you repeatedly used a sedative, hypnotic, or anxiolytic in situations in which it was physically hazardous, such as driving a car or operating a machine while impaired by sedative use?*

ix. Continued use despite awareness of physical or psychological problems: *Do you use sedatives, hypnotics, or anxiolytics even though you suspect, or even know, that your use creates or worsens problems with your mind and body?*

x. Tolerance as manifested by <u>either</u> of the following.

• Markedly increased amounts: *Do you find that in order to get intoxicated or achieve the desired effect of using sedatives, hypnotics, or anxiolytics, you need to consume much more than you used to?*

• Markedly diminished effects: *If you use the same amount of a sedative, hypnotic, or anxiolytic as you used to, do you find that it has a lot less effect on you than it used to?*

xi. Withdrawal as manifested by <u>either</u> of the following.

• Characteristic sedative, hypnotic, or anxiolytic withdrawal syndrome: *When you stop using sedatives, hypnotics, or anxiolytics, do you undergo withdrawal?*

• The same or a closely related substance is taken to relieve or avoid withdrawal symptoms: *Have you ever taken sedatives, hypnotics, anxiolytics, or another substance to prevent withdrawal?*

b. Modifiers

i. Specifiers

• In early remission
• In sustained remission
• In a controlled environment

ii. Severity

- Mild: Use when two or three criteria are present.
- Moderate: Use when four or five criteria are present.
- Severe: Use when six or more criteria are present.

c. Alternative: If a person experiences problems associated with the use of a sedative, hypnotic, or anxiolytic that are not classifiable as sedative, hypnotic, or anxiolytic use disorder; sedative, hypnotic, or anxiolytic intoxication; sedative, hypnotic, or anxiolytic withdrawal; sedative, hypnotic, or anxiolytic intoxication delirium; sedative, hypnotic, or anxiolytic withdrawal delirium; sedative-, hypnotic-, or anxiolytic-induced major or mild neurocognitive disorder; sedative-, hypnotic-, or anxiolytic-induced psychotic disorder; sedative-, hypnotic-, or anxiolytic-induced bipolar disorder; sedative-, hypnotic-, or anxiolytic-induced depressive disorder; sedative-, hypnotic-, or anxiolytic-induced anxiety disorder; sedative-, hypnotic-, or anxiolytic-induced sexual dysfunction; or sedative-, hypnotic-, or anxiolytic-induced sleep disorder, consider unspecified sedative-, hypnotic-, or anxiolytic-related disorder (see DSM-5, p. 560).

17. Sedative, Hypnotic, or Anxiolytic Intoxication

a. Inclusion: Requires <u>one</u> of the following signs shortly after sedative, hypnotic, or anxiolytic use.

i. Slurred speech
ii. Incoordination
iii. Unsteady gait
iv. Nystagmus
v. Impairment in cognition (i.e., attention or memory)
vi. Stupor or coma

b. Inclusion: Requires clinically significant problematic behavioral or psychological changes. *Since you began this episode of sedative, hypnotic, or anxiolytic use, have you observed any significant changes in your thoughts or behaviors? Have you done problematic things, or thought problematic thoughts, that you would not have without the sedative, hypnotic, or anxiolytic?*

c. Exclusion: If the symptoms are attributable to another medical condition or better explained by another mental disorder, including intoxication with another sub-stance, do not make the diagnosis.

18. Sedative, Hypnotic, or Anxiolytic Withdrawal

   a. Inclusion: Requires at least <u>two</u> of the following symptoms, developing within several hours to a few days after ceasing (or reducing) sedative, hypnotic, or anxiolytic use that has been heavy and prolonged.

      i. Autonomic hyperactivity
      ii. Hand tremor
      iii. Insomnia: *Over the last couple of days, have you found it more difficult than usual to get to sleep or to stay asleep?*
      iv. Nausea or vomiting: *Over the last couple of days, have you felt sick to your stomach, felt nauseated, or even vomited?*
      v. Transient visual, tactile, or auditory hallucinations or illusions: *Over the last couple of days, have you had any experiences where you worried that your mind was playing tricks on you, like seeing, hearing, or feeling things that other people could not?*
      vi. Psychomotor agitation
      vii. Anxiety: *Over the last couple of days, have you felt more worried or anxious than usual?*
      viii. Grand mal seizures

   b. Exclusion: If the symptoms are attributable to another medical condition or better explained by another mental disorder, including intoxication with or withdrawal from another substance, do not make the diagnosis.

   c. Modifiers

      i. Specifiers

         • With perceptual disturbances: Use when hallucinations occur with intact reality testing or when auditory, visual, or tactile illusions occur in the absence of delirium.

   d. Alternative: If a person experiences problems associated with the use of a sedative, hypnotic, or anxiolytic that are not classifiable as a sedative-, hypnotic-, or anxiolytic-related disorder, consider unspecified sedative-, hypnotic-, or anxiolytic-related disorder (see DSM-5, p. 560)

19. Stimulant Use Disorder

a. Inclusion: Requires a problematic pattern of stimulant use leading to clinically significant impairment or distress as manifested by at least <u>two</u> of the following in a 12-month period.

   i. Using more stimulants over a longer period than intended: *When you use stimulants, do you find that you use more, or for a longer time, than you planned to?*

   ii. Persistent desire or unsuccessful effort to reduce stimulant use: *Do you want to cut back or stop using stimulants? Have you ever tried and failed to cut back or stop using stimulants?*

   iii. Great deal of time spent: *Do you spend a great deal of your time obtaining stimulants, using stimulants, or recovering from your stimulant use?*

   iv. Cravings: *Do you experience strong desires or cravings to use stimulants?*

   v. Failure to fulfill major role obligations: *Have you repeatedly failed to fulfill major obligations at work, home, or school because of your stimulant use?*

   vi. Continued use despite awareness of interpersonal or social problems: *Do you use stimulants even though you suspect, or even know, that your use creates or worsens interpersonal or social problems?*

   vii. Giving up activities for stimulants: *Are there important social, occupational, or recreational activities that you have given up or reduced because of your stimulant use?*

   viii. Use in hazardous situations: *Have you repeatedly used stimulants in situations in which it was physically hazardous, such as driving a car or operating a machine while intoxicated?*

   ix. Continued use despite awareness of physical or psychological problems: *Do you use stimulants even though you suspect, or even know, that it creates or worsens problems with your mind and body?*

   x. Tolerance as manifested by <u>either</u> of the following. **Note:** This criterion is not met if taking stimulants as prescribed under medical supervision.

     • Markedly increased amounts: *Do you find that in order to get intoxicated or achieve the desired effect of using stimulants, you need to consume much more than you used to?*

- Markedly diminished effects: *If you use the same amount of a stimulant as you used to, do you find that it has a lot less effect on you than it used to?*

xi. Withdrawal as manifested by <u>either</u> of the following. **Note:** This criterion is not met if taking stimulants as prescribed under medical supervision.

- Characteristic stimulant withdrawal syndrome: *When you stop using stimulants, do you undergo withdrawal?*
- The same or a closely related substance is taken to relieve or avoid withdrawal symptoms: *Have you ever taken stimulants or another substance to prevent withdrawal?*

b. Modifiers

i. Specify stimulant

- Amphetamine-type substance
- Cocaine
- Other or unspecified stimulant

ii. Specifiers

- In early remission
- In sustained remission
- In a controlled environment

iii. Severity

- Mild: Use when two or three criteria are present.
- Moderate: Use when four or five criteria are present.
- Severe: Use when six or more criteria are present.

c. Alternative: If a person experiences problems associated with the use of stimulants that are not classifiable as stimulant use disorder, stimulant intoxication, stimulant withdrawal, stimulant intoxication delirium, stimulant-induced psychotic disorder, stimulant-induced bipolar disorder, stimulant-induced depressive disorder, stimulant-induced anxiety disorder, stimulant-induced sexual dysfunction, or stimulant-induced sleep disorder, consider unspecified stimulant-related disorder (see DSM-5, p. 570).

20. Stimulant Intoxication

    a. Inclusion: Requires at least <u>two</u> of the following signs shortly after stimulant use.

        i. Tachycardia or bradycardia
        ii. Pupillary dilation
        iii. Elevated or lowered blood pressure
        iv. Perspiration or chills: *Over the last couple of hours, have you experienced chills or been sweating more than usual?*
        v. Nausea or vomiting: *Over the last couple of hours, have you felt sick to your stomach, felt nauseated, or even vomited?*
        vi. Evidence of weight loss
        vii. Psychomotor agitation
        viii. Muscular weakness, respiratory depression, chest pain, or cardiac arrhythmias
        ix. Confusion, seizures, dyskinesias, dystonias, or coma

    b. Inclusion: Requires clinically significant problematic behavioral or psychological changes. *Since you began this episode of stimulant use, have you observed any significant changes in your thoughts or behaviors? Have you done problematic things, or thought problematic thoughts, that you would not have without the stimulant?*

    c. Exclusion: If the symptoms are due to another medical condition or better explained by another mental disorder, including intoxication with another substance, do not make the diagnosis.

    d. Modifiers

        i. Specifiers

           • With perceptual disturbances: Use when hallucinations occur with intact reality testing or when auditory, visual, or tactile illusions occur in the absence of delirium.

           • Amphetamine-type substance or cocaine

21. Stimulant Withdrawal

    a. Inclusion: Requires the following symptom, developing within hours to days of ceasing (or reducing) stimulant use that has been heavy and prolonged.

        i. Dysphoric mood: *Over the last few hours or days, have you felt much more down or depressed than usual?*

b. Inclusion: Also requires at least <u>two</u> of the following symptoms.

    i. Fatigue: *Over the last few hours or days, have you felt extremely sleepy or tired?*

    ii. Vivid, unpleasant dreams: *Over the last few hours or days, have you experienced unusually vivid, unpleasant dreams?*

    iii. Insomnia or hypersomnia: *Over the last few hours or days, have you found it more difficult than usual to get to sleep and to stay asleep? Alternatively, have you found that you have been sleeping much more than usual?*

    iv. Increased appetite: *Over the last few hours or days, have you desired food much more than usual?*

    v. Psychomotor retardation or agitation

c. Exclusion: If the symptoms are attributable to another medical condition or better explained by another mental disorder, including intoxication with or withdrawal from another substance, do not make the diagnosis.

d. Modifiers

    i. Amphetamine-type substance or cocaine

e. Alternative: If a person experiences problems associated with the use of a stimulant that are not classifiable as a stimulant-related disorder, consider unspecified stimulant-related disorder (see DSM-5, p. 570).

22. Tobacco Use Disorder

a. Inclusion: Requires a problematic pattern of tobacco use leading to clinically significant impairment or distress as manifested by at least <u>two</u> of the following in a 12-month period.

    i. Using more tobacco over a longer period than intended: *When you use tobacco, do you find that you use more, or for a longer time, than you planned to?*

    ii. Persistent desire or unsuccessful effort to reduce tobacco use: *Do you want to cut back or stop using tobacco? Have you ever tried and failed to cut back or stop using tobacco?*

    iii. Great deal of time spent: *Do you spend a great deal of your time obtaining tobacco, using tobacco, or recovering from your tobacco use?*

    iv. Cravings: *Do you experience strong desires or cravings to use tobacco?*

v. Failure to fulfill major role obligations: *Have you repeatedly failed to fulfill major obligations at work, home, or school because of your tobacco use?*

vi. Continued use despite awareness of interpersonal or social problems: *Do you use tobacco even though you suspect, or even know, that your use creates or worsens interpersonal or social problems?*

vii. Giving up activities for tobacco: *Are there important social, occupational, or recreational activities that you have given up or reduced because of your tobacco use?*

viii. Use in hazardous situations: *Have you repeatedly used tobacco in situations in which it was physically hazardous, like smoking in bed?*

ix. Continued use despite awareness of physical or psychological problems: *Do you use tobacco even though you suspect, or even know, that it creates or worsens problems with your mind and body?*

x. Tolerance as manifested by <u>either</u> of the following.

- Markedly increased amounts: *Do you find that in order to get the desired effect of tobacco, you need to use much more than you used to?*
- Markedly diminished effects: *If you use the same amount of tobacco as you used to, do you find that it has a lot less effect on you than it used to?*

xi. Withdrawal as manifested by <u>either</u> of the following.

- Characteristic tobacco withdrawal syndrome: *When you stop using tobacco, do you undergo withdrawal?*
- The same substance is taken to relieve or avoid withdrawal symptoms: *Have you ever used tobacco to avoid or relieve symptoms of tobacco withdrawal?*

b. Modifiers

i. Specifiers

- In early remission
- In sustained remission
- On maintenance therapy
- In a controlled environment

ii. Severity

- Mild: Use when two or three criteria are present.
- Moderate: Use when four or five criteria are present.
- Severe: Use when six or more criteria are present.

23. Tobacco Withdrawal

   a. Inclusion: Requires at least <u>four</u> of the following symptoms, developing within 24 hours of ceasing (or reducing) tobacco use that has been daily for at least several weeks.

      i. Irritability, frustration, or anger: *Over the last 24 hours, have you felt more irritable, frustrated, or angry than usual?*

      ii. Anxiety: *Over the last 24 hours, have you felt more worried or anxious than usual?*

      iii. Difficulty concentrating: *Over the last 24 hours, have you had difficulty staying focused on a task or activity?*

      iv. Increased appetite: *Over the last 24 hours, have you desired food more than usual?*

      v. Restlessness: *Over the last 24 hours, have you felt less able to remain at rest than usual?*

      vi. Depressed mood: *Over the last 24 hours, have you been feeling more down or depressed than usual?*

      vii. Insomnia: *Over the last 24 hours, have you found it more difficult than usual to get to sleep or to stay asleep?*

   b. Exclusion: If the symptoms are attributable to another medical condition or better explained by another mental disorder, including intoxication with or withdrawal from another substance, do not make the diagnosis.

   c. Alternative: If a person experiences problems associated with the use of tobacco that are not classifiable as a tobacco-related disorder, consider unspecified tobacco-related disorder (see DSM-5, p. 577).

24. Other (or Unknown) Substance Use Disorder

   a. Inclusion: Requires a problematic pattern of use of an intoxicating substance not able to be classified within the other substance categories above, leading to clinically significant impairment or distress as manifested by at least <u>two</u> of the following in a 12-month period.

      i. Taking more of the substance over a longer period than intended: *When you use the substance, do you find that you use it more often, or for a longer time, than you planned to?*

      ii. Persistent desire or unsuccessful effort to reduce substance use: *Do you want to cut back or stop using the substance? Have you ever tried and failed to cut back or stop using the substance?*

iii. Great deal of time spent: *Do you spend a great deal of your time obtaining or using the substance or recovering from your substance use?*

iv. Cravings: *Do you experience strong desires or cravings to use the substance?*

v. Failure to fulfill major role obligations: *Have you repeatedly failed to fulfill major obligations at work, home, or school because of your substance use?*

vi. Continued use despite awareness of interpersonal or social problems: *Do you use the substance even though you suspect, or even know, that it creates or worsens interpersonal or social problems?*

vii. Giving up activities for the substance: *Are there important social, occupational, or recreational activities that you have given up or reduced because of your substance use?*

viii. Use in hazardous situations: *Have you repeatedly used the substance in situations in which it was physically hazardous, such as driving a car or operating a machine while intoxicated?*

ix. Continued use despite awareness of physical or psychological problems: *Do you use the substance even though you suspect, or even know, that it creates or worsens problems with your mind and body?*

x. Tolerance as manifested by <u>either</u> of the following.

- Markedly increased amounts: *Do you find that in order to get intoxicated or achieve the desired effect of substance use, you need to consume much more of the substance than you used to?*
- Markedly diminished effects: *If you use the same amount of the substance as you used to, do you find that it has a lot less effect on you than it used to?*

xi. Withdrawal as manifested by <u>either</u> of the following.

- Characteristic withdrawal syndrome for the substance: *When you stop using the substance, do you undergo withdrawal?*
- The same or a closely related substance is taken to relieve or avoid withdrawal symptoms: *Have you ever taken the substance or another substance to prevent withdrawal?*

b. Modifiers

 i. Specifiers

 • In early remission
 • In sustained remission
 • In a controlled environment

 ii. Severity

 • Mild: Use when two or three symptoms are present.
 • Moderate: Use when four or five symptoms are present.
 • Severe: Use when six or more symptoms are present.

c. Alternatives

 i. If a person experiences problems associated with use of the substance that are not classifiable as other (or unknown) substance use disorder, other (or unknown) substance intoxication, or other (or unknown) substance withdrawal, consider unspecified other (or unknown) substance–related disorder (see DSM-5, p. 585).

25. Other (or Unknown) Substance Intoxication

a. Inclusion: Development of a reversible substance-specific syndrome attributable to recent ingestion of (or exposure to) a substance that is not listed elsewhere or is unknown.

b. Inclusion: Requires clinically significant problematic behavioral or psychological changes. *Since you began this episode of substance use, have you observed any significant changes in your behavior, mood, or judgment? Have you done problematic things, or thought problematic thoughts, that you would not have if you were not using the substance?*

c. Exclusion: If the symptoms are due to another medical condition or are better explained by another mental disorder, including intoxication with another substance, do not make the diagnosis.

26. Other (or Unknown) Substance Withdrawal

a. Inclusion: Development of a substance-specific syndrome shortly after the cessation of (or reduction in) use of the substance that has been heavy and prolonged.

b. Inclusion: Requires clinically significant distress or impairment in social, occupational, or other important areas of functioning.

c. Exclusion: If the symptoms are due to another medical condition or are better explained by another mental disorder, including withdrawal from another substance, do not make the diagnosis.

27. Gambling Disorder

a. Inclusion: Requires persistent, recurrent problematic gaming that leads to clinically significant impairment or distress, lasting at least 12 months, as indicated by at least <u>four</u> of the following symptoms.

    i. Escalates spending on gambling: *Do you find that it takes increasing amounts of money to get the excitement you want from gambling?*

    ii. Is irritable when quitting: *When you try to reduce or quit gambling, are you irritable or restless?*

    iii. Is unable to quit: *Have you unsuccessfully tried to reduce or quit gambling on several occasions?*

    iv. Is preoccupied: *Are you preoccupied with gambling?*

    v. Gambles when distressed: *When you are feeling anxious, down, or helpless, do you gamble?*

    vi. Chases losses: *After you lose money, do you return another day to try to get even?*

    vii. Lies: *Do you lie to conceal how much you gamble?*

    viii. Loses relationships: *Have you lost a relationship, job, or opportunity because of your gambling?*

    ix. Borrows money: *Do you have to rely on other people for money to cover desperate financial situations caused by gambling?*

b. Exclusion: If the gambling behavior is better accounted for by a manic episode, do not make the diagnosis.

c. Modifiers

    i. Course

        • Episodic: Meeting diagnostic criteria at more than one time point, with symptoms subsiding between periods of gambling disorder for at least several months

        • Persistent: Experiencing continuous symptoms to meet diagnostic criteria for multiple years

- In early remission
- In sustained remission

ii. Severity

- Mild: Use when four or five criteria are met.
- Moderate: Use when six or seven criteria are met.
- Severe: Use when eight or nine criteria are met.

Neurocognitive Disorders

DSM-5 pp. 591–643

Screening questions: Use Mini-Mental State Examination (MMSE).

- If a person is disoriented, proceed to delirium criteria.
- If a person is oriented but experiencing cognitive difficulties, ask: *Are you able to live as independently as you used to? For example, can you cook like you used to, and keep track of your medications and your finances like you used to?*
- If a person answers yes, proceed to mild neurocognitive disorder criteria.
- If a person, or his caregiver, answers no, proceed to major neurocognitive disorder criteria.

1. Delirium

    a. Inclusion: Requires the presence of all <u>three</u> of the following disturbances, which are usually assessed by means of the examination, especially the MMSE, rather than through diagnostic questions.

        i. Disturbance in attention and awareness as manifested by reduced ability to direct, focus, sustain, and shift attention
        ii. Disturbance that represents an acute change from baseline and that developed over a short period of time (hours to days), and with severity that tends to fluctuate during the day
        iii. Change in cognition, such as memory deficit, disorientation, language disturbance, visuospatial ability, or perception

    b. Exclusions

        i. If the change in cognition is better accounted for by a preexisting, established, or evolving neurocognitive disorder, do not make the diagnosis.
        ii. If the disturbance in cognition occurs in the context of a severely reduced level of arousal, such as coma, do not make the diagnosis.
        iii. If the disturbance in cognition is a direct physiological consequence of another medical condition, substance intoxication or withdrawal, or exposure

to a toxin, or is due to multiple etiologies, do not make the diagnosis.

c. Modifiers

    i. Subtypes

- Substance intoxication delirium: Use when inclusion criteria (i) and (iii) above predominate.
- Substance withdrawal delirium: Use when inclusion criteria (i) and (iii) above predominate.
- Medication-induced delirium: Use when inclusion criteria (ii) and (iii) arise as a side effect of a medication taken as prescribed.
- Delirium due to another medical condition
- Delirium due to multiple etiologies

    ii. Specifiers

- Course
  - Acute: Lasting a few hours or days
  - Persistent: Lasting weeks or months
- Descriptive features
  - Hyperactive
  - Hypoactive
  - Mixed level of activity

d. Alternative: If you are unable to determine why a person is experiencing delirium, or if his delirium is subsyndromal, consider unspecified delirium (see DSM-5, p. 602). If you wish to communicate the specific reason a person's symptoms do not meet full criteria for delirium, consider other specified delirium (see DSM-5, p. 602). An example is attenuated delirium syndrome.

2. Major Neurocognitive Disorder

a. Inclusion: Requires evidence of significant cognitive decline from a previous level of performance in one or more cognitive domains based on <u>both</u> of the following, which are usually assessed using the examination, especially the MMSE, rather than through diagnostic questions.

    i. A person's self-concern, or the concern of a knowledgeable informant or the clinician, that a significant cognitive decline has occurred

    ii. A substantial impairment in cognitive performance, preferably documented by standardized neuropsychological testing or, in its absence, another quantified clinical assessment

b. Inclusion: Also, the cognitive deficits interfere with independence in everyday activities.

c. Exclusion: If the cognitive impairments occur exclusively while the patient is delirious or are primarily the result of another mental disorder, do not make the diagnosis.

d. Modifiers

   i. Subtypes: Specify whether due to:

   • Alzheimer's disease: Characteristically associated with an insidious onset and gradual progression, in which memory impairment is an early and prominent feature. Requires exclusion of other known neurocognitive disorders. (Full criteria are in DSM-5, pp. 611–612.)

   • Frontotemporal lobar degeneration: Requires evidence for the characteristic impairments associated with behavioral or language variants. The behavioral variant can include prominent decline in social cognition and/or executive abilities; disinhibition; apathy or inertia; loss of sympathy or empathy; perseverative, stereotyped, or compulsive/ritualistic behavior; and hyperorality and dietary changes. The language variant includes prominent decline in language ability, in the form of speech production, word finding, object naming, grammar, or word comprehension. In both variants, learning, memory, and perceptual motor function are relatively spared. Requires the exclusion of another neurocognitive disorder. (Full criteria are in DSM-5, pp. 614–615.)

   • Lewy body disease: Requires evidence of fluctuating cognition with pronounced variations in attention and alertness, recurrent visual hallucinations that are typically well formed and detailed, and spontaneous features of parkinsonism with onset of motor symptoms at least 1 year later than the cognitive impairment. Requires the exclusion of another neurocognitive disorder. (Full criteria are in DSM-5, pp. 618–619.)

- Vascular disease: Requires evidence of cerebro-vascular disease and exclusion of other known neurocognitive disorders. Deficits in the speed of information processing, complex attention, or frontal-executive functioning are characteristic. Onset is temporally related to one or more cerebrovascular events. (Full criteria are in DSM-5, p. 621.)

- Traumatic brain injury: Requires an impact to the head or other rapid displacement of the brain within the skull that results in <u>one</u> or more of the following: loss of consciousness, posttraumatic amnesia, disorientation and confusion, or neurological signs. The cognitive deficits present immediately following the injury or after recovery of consciousness and persist past the acute post-injury period (i.e., for at least 1 week). (Full criteria are in DSM-5, p. 624.)

- Substance/medication use: Requires presumptive evidence of an etiological relationship between past or present substance use and cognitive deficits. A person must have used a substance or medication for a duration and extent capable of producing the neurocognitive impairment. Requires the exclusion of another medical condition or mental disorder or current intoxication or withdrawal. (Full criteria are in DSM-5, pp. 627–629.)

- HIV infection: Requires documented infection with HIV. Symptoms cannot be better explained by secondary brain diseases like progressive multifocal leukoencephalopathy or cryptococcal meningitis. Requires the exclusion of another neurocognitive disorder. (Full criteria are in DSM-5, p. 632.)

- Prion disease: Requires evidence that the neurocognitive disorder is due to a prion disease. Requires the presence of motor features of prion disease or biomarker evidence. Requires the exclusion of cognitive deficits due to delirium or another mental disorder. (Full criteria are in DSM-5, pp. 634–635.)

- Parkinson's disease: Requires the established presence of Parkinson's disease and the insidious onset and gradual progression of impairing cognitive deficits. (Full criteria are in DSM-5, pp. 636–637.)

- Huntington's disease: Requires the presence of clinically established Huntington's disease or evidence of risk for the disease based on family history or genetic testing, and the insidious onset and gradual progression of impairing cognitive deficits. (Full criteria are in DSM-5, pp. 638–639.)
- Another medical condition: Requires evidence that the neurocognitive disorder is due to another medical condition. Requires the exclusion of cognitive deficits due to delirium or another mental disorder. (Full criteria are in DSM-5, p. 641.)
- Multiple etiologies: Requires evidence from the history, physical examination, or laboratory findings that the neurocognitive disorder is the pathophysiological consequence of more than one etiological process, excluding substances. Requires the exclusion of cognitive deficits due to delirium or another mental disorder. (Full criteria are in DSM-5, p. 642.)
- Unspecified: Can be used in the event of a subthreshold syndrome, an atypical presentation, an uncertain etiology, or a specific syndrome not listed in DSM-5. (See DSM-5, p. 643.)

ii. Specifiers

- Without behavioral disturbance
- With behavioral disturbance

iii. Severity

- Mild: Use when some difficulties with instrumental activities of daily living are present.
- Moderate: Use when difficulties with basic activities of daily living are present.
- Severe: Use when a person is fully dependent on other people.

3. Mild Neurocognitive Disorder

a. Inclusion: Requires evidence of significant cognitive decline from a previous level of performance in one or more cognitive domains based on <u>both</u> of the following, which are usually assessed using the examination, especially the MMSE, rather than through diagnostic questions.

    i. A person's self-concern, or the concern of a knowledgeable informant or the clinician, that a significant cognitive decline has occurred

    ii. A substantial impairment in cognitive performance, preferably documented by standardized neuropsychological testing or, in its absence, another quantified clinical assessment

b. Inclusion: Also, the cognitive deficits do not interfere with capacity for independence in everyday activities (but greater effort, compensatory strategies, or accommodation may be required).

c. Exclusion: If the cognitive impairments occur exclusively while the patient is delirious or are primarily the result of another mental disorder, do not make the diagnosis.

d. Modifiers

    i. Subtypes (see full descriptions in major neurocognitive disorder above): Specify whether due to:

- Alzheimer's disease
- Frontotemporal lobar degeneration
- Lewy body disease
- Vascular disease
- Traumatic brain injury
- Substance/medication use
- HIV infection
- Prion disease
- Parkinson's disease
- Huntington's disease
- Another medical condition
- Multiple etiologies
- Unspecified

    ii. Specifiers

- Without behavioral disturbance
- With behavioral disturbance

Personality Disorders

DSM-5 pp. 645–684

Screening questions: *When anyone reflects on their life, they can identify patterns—characteristic thoughts, moods, and actions— that began when they were a young person and have subsequently occurred in many personal and social situations. Thinking about your own life, can you identify patterns like that which have caused you significant problems with your friends or family, at work, or in another setting?*

    If yes, ask: *When you think about these characteristic patterns of behavior that began when you were a young person, can you recognize enduring patterns in the way you perceive yourself and other people, the ways you respond emotionally to exciting or difficult circumstances, the ways you interact with other people, or your ability to control your impulses and urges?*

    If yes, ask: *When you look over your life, can you see that one or more of the following ways of being has been relatively stable over time?*

- *Distrusting other people and suspecting them of being mean*
- *Feeling disconnected from close relationships and preferring not to express much emotion*
- *Feeling uncomfortable in close relationships and preferring activities that many other people consider unusual or eccentric*
- *Disregarding the rights of other people without concern for how it affects them*
- *Experiencing yourself, your mood, and your relationships as constantly changing*
- *Being more emotional and desiring more attention than other people*
- *Sensing that you are much more accomplished or deserving than other people*
- *Avoiding other people because you feel inferior or fear they will criticize or reject you*
- *Wanting so much for someone to take care of you that you become submissive or clingy and repeatedly fear they will separate from you*
- *Focusing on getting things rightly ordered, perfect, or in control*

- If distrust and suspiciousness of others predominates, proceed to paranoid personality disorder criteria.

- If detachment and restricted range of emotions predominate, proceed to schizoid personality disorder criteria.
- If discomfort in close relationships and eccentric behavior predominate, proceed to schizotypal personality disorder criteria.
- If disregard for the rights of other people predominates, proceed to antisocial personality disorder criteria.
- If instability in relationships, self-image, and affects predominates, proceed to borderline personality disorder criteria.
- If excessive emotionality and attention seeking predominate, proceed to histrionic personality disorder criteria.
- If grandiosity and need for admiration predominate, proceed to narcissistic personality disorder criteria.
- If social inhibition and feelings of inadequacy predominate, proceed to avoidant personality disorder criteria.
- If a need to be taken care of predominates, proceed to dependent personality disorder criteria.
- If preoccupation with orderliness, perfectionism, and control predominates, proceed to obsessive-compulsive personality disorder criteria.

1. Paranoid Personality Disorder

   a. Inclusion: Requires a pervasive pattern of distrust and suspiciousness of others such that their motives are interpreted as malevolent, as indicated by at least <u>four</u> of the following manifestations.

      i. Suspects exploitation or harm: *Do you frequently suspect that other people are exploiting, harming, or deceiving you, even when you have limited evidence for these suspicions?*

      ii. Preoccupied with doubts: *Do you find that thinking about whether or not the people in your life are loyal or trustworthy dominates your thoughts?*

      iii. Reluctant to confide: *Are you often reluctant to tell someone about a personal or private matter because you fear they will use the information to harm you?*

      iv. Reads hidden meanings: *Do other people often say things or do things to demean or threaten you?*

      v. Persistently bears grudges: *When someone insults, injures, or slights you, do you find it very hard to forgive? Do you usually bear grudges?*

      vi. Perceives character attacks: *Do you find that other people often say or do things to attack your character or reputation? Do you counterattack or react angrily to people?*

    vii. Suspects infidelity: *When you are involved in a relationship, do you repeatedly suspect your partner of being unfaithful to you, without having any evidence?*

  b. Exclusion: If the disturbance occurs exclusively in the course of a psychotic disorder, or a bipolar or depressive disorder with psychotic features, or is a physiological effect of another medical condition, do not make the diagnosis.

2. Schizoid Personality Disorder

  a. Inclusion: Requires a pervasive pattern of detachment from social relationships and a restricted range of expression of emotions in interpersonal settings, as indicated by at least <u>four</u> of the following manifestations.

    i. Neither desires nor enjoys close relationships: *Do you find that you neither desire to be nor enjoy being close to other people, including your family?*

    ii. Chooses solitary activities: *When you have a choice, do you almost always choose activities that you can do alone, without other people?*

    iii. Little interest in sexual experiences with others: *Would it be okay with you if you lived the rest of your life without romantic or sexual experiences with other people?*

    iv. Takes pleasure in few activities: *Do you find that very few activities bring you pleasure or enjoyment?*

    v. Lacks close friends and confidants: *Other than your immediate family, do you find that you do not have close friends or people with whom you share personal matters or secrets?*

    vi. Appears indifferent to praise or criticism: *When other people praise or criticize you, do you find that it does not affect you?*

    vii. Shows emotional coldness or detachment: *Do you rarely experience strong emotions like anger or joy? Do you rarely reciprocate gestures or facial expressions like smiles or nods?*

  b. Exclusion: If the disturbance occurs exclusively in the course of a psychotic disorder, a bipolar or depressive disorder with psychotic features, or autism spectrum disorder, or is a physiological effect of another medical condition, do not make the diagnosis.

3. Schizotypal Personality Disorder

   a. Inclusion: Requires a pervasive pattern of social and interpersonal deficits marked by acute discomfort with, and reduced capacity for, close relationships as well as by cognitive or perceptual distortions or eccentricities, as indicated by at least <u>five</u> of the following manifestations.

      i. Ideas of reference: *Does it often feel as though other people are talking about you or watching you?*

      ii. Odd beliefs or magical thinking: *Are you very superstitious? Are you preoccupied with paranormal or magical phenomena? Do you have special powers to sense events before they happen or to read the thoughts of other people?*

      iii. Unusual perceptual experiences: *Do you sometimes have the sense that another person, whom other people cannot see, is present and speaking with you?*

      iv. Odd thinking and speech: *Do other people ever tell you that the things you say, or the way you say them, are unusual or even inappropriate?*

      v. Suspiciousness or paranoia: *Do you frequently suspect that other people are exploiting, harming, or deceiving you?*

      vi. Inappropriate or constricted affect: *Do you notice that your emotional experiences and expressions stay within a narrow range and do not change much over time? Have other people told you that you do not respond to emotionally provocative situations as they expect?*

      vii. Odd or eccentric appearance or behavior: *Do other people ever respond to you as if your behavior or appearance was odd or bizarre?*

      viii. Lacks close friends and confidants: *Other than your immediate family, do you find that you do not have close friends or people with whom you share personal matters or secrets?*

      ix. Excessive social anxiety: *Are you usually worried or anxious in social settings, especially when around unfamiliar people?*

   b. Exclusion: If the disturbance occurs exclusively in the course of a psychotic disorder, a bipolar or depressive disorder with psychotic features, or an autism spectrum disorder, do not make the diagnosis.

4. Antisocial Personality Disorder

   a. Inclusion: Requires a pervasive pattern of disregard for and violation of the rights of others, as indicated by at least <u>three</u> of the following manifestations.

      i. Repeatedly performing acts that are grounds for arrest: *Have you repeatedly destroyed or stolen the property of other people, harassed other people, or done other things that could have gotten you arrested?*

      ii. Deceitfulness: *Do you often misrepresent yourself by claiming accomplishments, qualities, or identities that are not your own? Do you often deceive other people for pleasure or financial gain?*

      iii. Impulsivity: *Do you often struggle to formulate and follow a plan? Do you often act on the spur of the moment, without a plan or consideration of the consequences?*

      iv. Aggressiveness resulting in assaults: *Are you often so grumpy or irritable that you frequently confront or even attack other people? Have you ever attacked someone or been in physical fights that did not begin as self-defense?*

      v. Reckless disregard for safety: *Do you often engage in dangerous, risky, and potentially self-damaging activities with little thought to the consequences for yourself or others?*

      vi. Consistent irresponsibility: *When you enter into agreements or make promises, do you often disregard and fail to follow through on your commitments? When you have familial obligations and financial debts, do you often disregard them?*

      vii. Lack of remorse: *Are you rarely concerned about the feelings, needs, or suffering of other people? If you have ever hurt or mistreated someone else, did you feel very little regret or remorse after doing so?*

   b. Inclusion: Evidence of conduct disorder with onset before the age of 15 years.

   c. Exclusion: If the disturbance occurs exclusively in the course of a psychotic or bipolar disorder, do not make the diagnosis.

5. Borderline Personality Disorder

   a. Inclusion: Requires a pervasive pattern of instability of interpersonal relationships, self-image, and affects, and marked impulsivity, as indicated by at least <u>five</u> of the following manifestations.

i. Frantic efforts to avoid abandonment: *When you sense that someone close to you is going to abandon you, do you undertake emotional or even frantic efforts to keep them from leaving you?*

ii. Unstable interpersonal relationships: *Are most of your close relationships intense and unstable? Do you alternate between feeling as though the people in your life are really good and really bad?*

iii. Identity disturbance: *Do you have a very unstable or poorly developed sense of who you are? Do your aspirations, goals, opinions, and values change suddenly and frequently?*

iv. Self-damaging impulsivity in at least two areas that are not suicidal or self-mutilating behavior: *Do you often act on the spur of the moment, without a plan or consideration for the outcome? Do you frequently engage in dangerous, risky, and potentially self-damaging activities without regard to their consequences?*

v. Parasuicidal or suicidal behavior: *Do you frequently threaten to harm yourself or even kill yourself? Have you made recurrent attempts to hurt, harm, or kill yourself?*

vi. Affective instability: *Are your emotions easily aroused or intense? Do you often have intense feelings of sadness, annoyance, or worry that usually only last a few hours and never more than a few days?*

vii. Chronic emptiness: *Do you chronically feel empty?*

viii. Anger: *Do you often experience intense anger, often much stronger than the event or circumstance that triggered it, and frequently lose your temper?*

ix. Transient paranoia or dissociation: *At times of stress, do you ever feel like other people are conspiring against you or that you are an outside observer of your own mind, thoughts, feelings, and body?*

6. Histrionic Personality Disorder

   a. Inclusion: Requires a pervasive pattern of excessive emotionality and attention seeking, as indicated by at least <u>five</u> of the following manifestations.

      i. Uncomfortable when not the center of attention: *Do you usually feel uncomfortable or unappreciated when you are not the center of attention?*

ii. Seductive or provocative behavior: *Do you flirt with most of the people you meet, even if you are not attracted to them?*

iii. Shifting and shallow emotions: *When you express emotions or feelings, do they change rapidly? Have other people told you that your emotions seem to have little depth or to be insincere?*

iv. Uses appearance to draw attention: *Do you usually 'dress to impress,' spending your time and energy on your clothes and appearance so you can draw attention to yourself?*

v. Impressionistic and vague speech: *Do other people ever tell you that you have strong opinions but that they find it hard to understand the underlying reasons for your opinions?*

vi. Dramatic or exaggerated emotions: *Are you a very expressive or even dramatic person? Have your friends or family repeatedly told you that you embarrassed them with your public displays of emotion?*

vii. Suggestible: *Do you frequently change your opinions and feelings based on the people around you or the people you admire?*

viii. Considers relationships more intimate than they are: *Do you often feel close to people early in a relationship and share personal details of your life? Have you been hurt by relationships that you thought were more serious or intimate than the other person did?*

7. Narcissistic Personality Disorder

a. Inclusion: Requires a pervasive pattern of grandiosity (in fantasy or behavior), need for admiration, and lack of empathy, as indicated by at least <u>five</u> of the following manifestations.

i. Grandiose sense of self-importance: *Would you describe yourself and your accomplishments as so special and unique that they set you apart from your peers?*

ii. Preoccupied with fantasies of unlimited success: *When you imagine the life of your dreams, do you think a lot about having unlimited success, limitless power, unparalleled brilliance, remarkable beauty, or supreme love?*

iii. High-status understanding: *Are your abilities and needs so special that you feel as though you should associate only with gifted people or institutions? Do you feel that only unique or gifted people are capable of understanding you?*

    iv. Requires excessive admiration: *Do you often feel offended if people you respect do not give you the admiration you deserve?*

    v. Entitlement: *Do you often get annoyed or irritated when people do not follow your wishes or give you the treatment you deserve?*

    vi. Exploitative: *Are you good at getting people to do what you want? Do you ever take advantage of people to get the resources or privileges you deserve?*

    vii. Lacks empathy: *Do you find it hard to recognize or identify with the feelings and needs of other people?*

    viii. Envious: *Do other people really envy you or your life? Do you spend a lot of time envying other people or their lives?*

    ix. Arrogant behaviors or attitudes: *Have other people ever told you that you acted haughty, patronizing, or arrogant?*

8. Avoidant Personality Disorder

    a. Inclusion: Requires a pervasive pattern of social inhibition, feelings of inadequacy, and hypersensitivity to negative evaluations, as indicated by at least <u>four</u> of the following manifestations.

        i. Avoids occupational activities involving interpersonal contact: *Do you often avoid school or work activities that involve a lot of contact with other people because you fear they will criticize or reject you?*

        ii. Needs assurance before getting involved with other people: *Do you avoid making new friends unless you are certain they like you and accept you without criticism?*

        iii. Fear of being shamed limits intimate relationships: *In your close relationships, are you usually cautious or restrained because you fear being shamed or ridiculed?*

        iv. Preoccupied with criticism in social situations: *In social situations, do you spend a great deal of time worrying that other people will criticize or reject you?*

        v. Inadequacy inhibits interpersonal situations: *In new relationships, are you usually shy, quiet, or inhibited because you fear that other people will find you inadequate or unsuitable?*

     vi. Negative self-perception: *Do you perceive yourself to be socially inept, personally unappealing, or inferior to others?*

    vii. Reluctant to take risks: *Are you usually reluctant to take personal risks or engage in any new activities because you fear you will be embarrassed?*

9. Dependent Personality Disorder

    a. Inclusion: Requires a pervasive and excessive need to be taken care of that leads to submissive and clinging behavior and fears of separation, as indicated by at least <u>five</u> of the following manifestations.

       i. Struggles to make everyday decisions without reassurance: *Do you struggle to make everyday decisions like what to eat or wear without advice and reassurance from other people?*

      ii. Needs others to assume responsibility: *Do you prefer to let someone else take responsibility for the major decisions in your life like where to live, the kind of work you do, and who you befriend?*

     iii. Struggles to disagree: *Do you find it really hard to disagree with the people you count on because you fear they will disapprove or withdraw their support of you?*

     iv. Struggles to initiate: *Do you usually lack the self-confidence to start a new project or do things independently?*

      v. Excessive lengths to obtain support: *Do you go to great lengths to receive care and support from other people, even volunteering to do things that you find unpleasant?*

     vi. Feels helpless when alone: *When you are alone, do you often feel uncomfortable or even helpless because you fear being unable to care for yourself?*

    vii. Urgently seeks relationships: *After a close relationship ends, do you urgently seek another relationship in which you can receive the care and support you need?*

   viii. Preoccupied with fears of being alone: *Do you spend a great deal of time worrying about being left alone with no one to care for you?*

10. Obsessive-Compulsive Personality Disorder

    a. Inclusion: Requires a pervasive pattern of preoccupation with orderliness, perfectionism, and mental and interpersonal control, at the expense of flexibility, openness, and efficiency, as indicated by at least <u>four</u> of the following manifestations.

    i.   Preoccupation with order interferes with the point of the activity: *Do you often find that you are so focused on the details, rules, lists, order, organization, or schedules for an activity that you lose the essential point of the activity?*

    ii.   Perfectionism interferes with task completion: *Are you often unable to complete projects because you cannot meet the high standards you set for yourself?*

    iii.   Devoted to work at the expense of friendships: *Do you devote so much time and energy to your work that you have little time for friendships or recreational activities? When you do participate in recreational activities, do you approach them as serious tasks that require organization and mastery?*

    iv.   Scrupulosity: *Do other people who share your cultural or religious identification ever tell you that they find you too strict or too concerned with not doing something wrong? Do you aspire to moral standards that are so high that it is difficult for you to realize your goals?*

    v.   Unable to discard worn-out objects: *Do you often find it hard to discard worn-out or worthless objects even when they have no sentimental value?*

    vi.   Reluctant to give up control of tasks: *Do you find it hard to work with other people or delegate tasks because you fear they will not do things the way you would?*

    vii.   Miserly: *Do you usually find it hard to spend money on yourself or other people? Do you maintain a standard of living well below what you can afford so you can save money for a catastrophe?*

    viii.   Rigidity: *Does your need to be right, or to not change your position, frequently make it difficult to make and maintain relationships with other people?*

11. Alternative:

    a.   If a person exhibits a persistent personality disturbance that represents a change from her previous characteristic personality pattern and there is evidence that the disturbance is the direct consequence of another medical condition, consider personality change due to another medical condition (full criteria and multiple specifiers are in DSM-5, p. 682). If the diagnosis is better explained by another mental disorder, occurs exclusively during an episode of delirium, or does not cause clinically significant distress or impairment, do not make the diagnosis.

b. If a person exhibits symptoms characteristic of a personality disorder that cause clinically significant distress or impairment but do not meet full criteria for a specific personality disorder, consider unspecified personality disorder (see DSM-5, p. 684). If you wish to communicate the specific reason that the presentation does not meet the criteria for a specific personality disorder, consider other specified personality disorder (see DSM-5, p. 684).

Paraphilic Disorders

DSM-5 pp. 685–705

Screening question: *Are there any particular urges, fantasies, or behaviors that repeatedly cause you to feel intensely aroused?*

If yes, ask: *Has satisfying these fantasies or urges put you or someone else at harm? OR Have you acted on these fantasies or urges with someone who did not want to be involved?*

- If yes, proceed to paraphilic disorder criteria.

1. Paraphilic Disorders

    a. Inclusion: Requires a paraphilia, which is any intense and persistent sexual interest other than sexual interest in genital stimulation with mature, consenting partners. However, the paraphilia must be intense and persistent for at least 6 months and must be currently causing distress or impairment in the individual, or entail personal harm or risk of harm to others, to qualify as a disorder.

        i. Paraphilia: *Different people are aroused by different fantasies. I am going to read a list of fantasies and would like you to tell me if you have frequent, recurrent fantasies, urges, or behaviors about any of these.*

            - Voyeuristic disorder: *Are you aroused by watching, or thinking about watching, other people when they are disrobing, naked, or engaged in sexual activity and do not know you are watching?*
            - Exhibitionistic disorder: *Are you aroused by the thought of exposing your genitals to a person who does not want to be exposed to them?*
            - Frotteuristic disorder: *Are you aroused by the thought of touching or rubbing against another person?*
            - Sexual masochism disorder: *Are you aroused by the thought of being humiliated, bound, beaten, or otherwise made to suffer?*
            - Sexual sadism disorder: *Are you aroused by the physical or psychological suffering of another person?*
            - Pedophilic disorder: *Are you aroused by sexual activity with prepubescent or pubescent children?*

- Fetishistic disorder: *Are you aroused by nonliving objects other than clothes used in cross-dressing or devices designed for genital stimulation? Are you aroused by specific nongenital body parts like feet, toes, or hair?*
- Transvestic disorder: *Are you aroused by cross-dressing?*

b. Exclusions

   i. For the diagnosis of voyeuristic disorder, the person experiencing the arousal and/or acting on the urges must be at least 18 years of age.

   ii. For the diagnosis of pedophilic disorder, the person must be at least 16 years of age and at least 5 years older than the child or children who are the object(s) of arousal.

   iii. For the diagnosis of fetishistic disorder, the object of arousal cannot include clothing used in cross-dressing or objects specifically designed for tactile genital stimulation, such as a vibrator.

c. Modifiers

   i. Course specifiers common to paraphilic disorders (do not apply to pedophilic disorder)

   - In a controlled environment
   - In full remission (no recurring behavior or distress or impairment for at least 5 years while in an uncontrolled environment)

   ii. Exhibitionistic disorder subtypes

   - Sexually aroused by exposing genitals to prepubertal children
   - Sexually aroused by exposing genitals to physically mature individuals
   - Sexually aroused by exposing genitals to prepubertal children and to physically mature individuals

   iii. Sexual masochism disorder specifier

   - With asphyxiophilia (i.e., sexually aroused by asphyxiation)

   iv. Pedophilic disorder subtypes

   - Exclusive type (attracted only to children)
   - Nonexclusive type

v. Pedophilic disorder specifiers

- Sexually attracted to males
- Sexually attracted to females
- Sexually attracted to both
- Limited to incest

vi. Fetishistic disorder specifiers

- Body part(s)
- Nonliving object(s)
- Other

vii. Transvestic disorder specifiers

- With fetishism (sexually aroused by fabrics, materials, or garments)
- With autogynephilia (sexually aroused by thought or image of self as female)

d. Alternatives: If a person endorses a paraphilia that is not included in this list, consider unspecified paraphilic disorder (see DSM-5, p. 705). If you wish to communicate the specific reason a person's presentation does not meet full criteria for a disorder above, consider other specified paraphilic disorder (see DSM-5, p. 705). DSM-5 includes a partial list of paraphilias that can occur within a paraphilic disorder: telephone scatologia disorder (obscene phone calls), necrophilic disorder (corpses), zoophilic disorder (animals), coprophilic disorder (feces), klismaphilic disorder (enemas), and urophilic disorder (urine).

Medication-Induced Movement Disorders and Other Adverse Effects of Medication

DSM-5 pp. 709–714

ICD-9-CM code	ICD-10-CM code	Description
332.1	G21.11	Neuroleptic-induced parkinsonism
332.1	G21.19	Other medication-induced parkinsonism
333.92	G21.0	Neuroleptic malignant syndrome
333.72	G24.02	Medication-induced acute dystonia
333.99	G25.71	Medication-induced acute akathisia
333.85	G24.01	Tardive dyskinesia
333.72	G24.09	Tardive dystonia
333.99	G25.71	Tardive akathisia
333.1	G25.1	Medication-induced postural tremor
333.99	G25.79	Other medication-induced movement disorder
		Antidepressant discontinuation syndrome
995.29	T43.205A	Initial encounter
995.29	T43.205D	Subsequent encounter
995.29	T43.205S	Sequelae
		Other adverse effect of medication
995.20	T50.905A	Initial encounter
995.20	T50.905D	Subsequent encounter
995.20	T50.905S	Sequelae

Other Conditions That May Be a Focus of Clinical Attention

DSM-5 pp. 715–727

DSM-5 includes other conditions and problems that may be a focus of clinical attention or that may otherwise affect the diagnosis, course, prognosis, or treatment of a patient's mental disorder. These conditions and problems include, but are not limited to, the psychosocial and environmental problems that were coded on Axis IV in DSM-IV-TR. The authors of DSM-5 provide a selected list of conditions and problems drawn from ICD-9-CM (usually V codes) and ICD-10-CM (usually Z codes). A condition or problem listed below may be coded if it is a reason for the current visit or helps to explain the need for a test, procedure, or treatment.

Conditions and problems from this list may also be included in the medical record as useful information on circumstances that may affect the patient's care, regardless of their relevance to the current visit. The conditions and problems listed in this chapter are not mental disorders. Their inclusion in DSM-5 is meant to draw attention to the scope of additional issues that are encountered in routine clinical practice and to provide a systematic listing that may be useful to clinicians in documenting these issues.

ICD-9-CM code	ICD-10-CM code	Description
V61.20	Z62.820	Parent-child relational problem
V61.8	Z62.891	Sibling relational problem
V61.8	Z62.29	Upbringing away from parents
V61.29	Z62.898	Child affected by parental relationship distress
V61.10	Z63.0	Relationship distress with spouse or intimate partner
V61.03	Z63.5	Disruption of family by separation or divorce
V61.8	Z63.8	High expressed emotion level within family
V62.82	Z63.4	Uncomplicated bereavement

ICD-9-CM code	ICD-10-CM code	Description
		Child physical abuse, confirmed
995.54	T74.12XA	Initial encounter
995.54	T74.12XD	Subsequent encounter
		Child physical abuse, suspected
995.54	T76.12XA	Initial encounter
995.54	T76.12XD	Subsequent encounter
		Other circumstances related to child physical abuse
V61.21	Z69.010	Encounter for mental health services for victim of child abuse by parent
V61.21	Z69.020	Encounter for mental health services for victim of nonparental child abuse
V15.41	Z62.810	Personal history (past history) of physical abuse in childhood
V61.22	Z69.011	Encounter for mental health services for perpetrator of parental child abuse
V62.83	Z69.021	Encounter for mental health services for perpetrator of nonparental child abuse
		Child sexual abuse, confirmed
995.53	T74.22XA	Initial encounter
995.53	T74.22XD	Subsequent encounter
		Child sexual abuse, suspected
995.53	T76.22XA	Initial encounter
995.53	T76.22XD	Subsequent encounter
		Other circumstances related to child sexual abuse
V61.21	Z69.010	Encounter for mental health services for victim of child sexual abuse by parent

ICD-9-CM code	ICD-10-CM code	Description
		Other circumstances related to child sexual abuse *(continued)*
V61.21	Z69.020	Encounter for mental health services for victim of nonparental child sexual abuse
V15.41	Z62.810	Personal history (past history) of sexual abuse in childhood
V61.22	Z69.011	Encounter for mental health services for perpetrator of parental child sexual abuse
V62.83	Z69.021	Encounter for mental health services for perpetrator of nonparental child sexual abuse
		Child neglect, confirmed
995.52	T74.02XA	Initial encounter
995.52	T74.02XD	Subsequent encounter
		Child neglect, suspected
995.52	T76.02XA	Initial encounter
995.52	T76.02XD	Subsequent encounter
		Other circumstances related to child neglect
V61.21	Z69.010	Encounter for mental health services for victim of child neglect by parent
V61.21	Z69.020	Encounter for mental health services for victim of nonparental child neglect
V15.42	Z62.812	Personal history (past history) of neglect in childhood
V61.22	Z69.011	Encounter for mental health services for perpetrator of parental child neglect
V62.83	Z69.021	Encounter for mental health services for perpetrator of nonparental child neglect

ICD-9-CM code	ICD-10-CM code	Description
		Child psychological abuse, confirmed
995.51	T74.32XA	Initial encounter
995.51	T74.32XD	Subsequent encounter
		Child psychological abuse, suspected
995.51	T76.32XA	Initial encounter
995.51	T76.32XD	Subsequent encounter
		Other circumstances related to child psychological abuse
V61.21	Z69.010	Encounter for mental health services for victim of child psychological abuse by parent
V61.21	Z69.020	Encounter for mental health services for victim of nonparental child psychological abuse
V15.42	Z62.811	Personal history (past history) of psychological abuse in childhood
V61.22	Z69.011	Encounter for mental health services for perpetrator of parental child psychological abuse
V62.83	Z69.021	Encounter for mental health services for perpetrator of nonparental child psychological abuse
		Spouse or partner violence, physical, confirmed
995.81	T74.11XA	Initial encounter
995.81	T74.11XD	Subsequent encounter
		Spouse or partner violence, physical, suspected
995.81	T76.11XA	Initial encounter
995.81	T76.11XD	Subsequent encounter

ICD-9-CM code	ICD-10-CM code	Description
		Other circumstances related to spouse or partner violence, physical
V61.11	Z69.11	Encounter for mental health services for victim of spouse or partner violence, physical
V15.41	Z91.410	Personal history (past history) of spouse or partner violence, physical
V61.12	Z69.12	Encounter for mental health services for perpetrator of spouse or partner violence, physical
		Spouse or partner violence, sexual, confirmed
995.83	T74.21XA	Initial encounter
995.83	T74.21XD	Subsequent encounter
		Spouse or partner violence, sexual, suspected
995.83	T76.21XA	Initial encounter
995.83	T76.21XD	Subsequent encounter
		Other circumstances related to spouse or partner violence, sexual
V61.11	Z69.81	Encounter for mental health services for victim of spouse or partner violence, sexual
V15.41	Z91.410	Personal history (past history) of spouse or partner violence, sexual
V61.12	Z69.12	Encounter for mental health services for perpetrator of spouse or partner violence, sexual

ICD-9-CM code	ICD-10-CM code	Description
		Spouse or partner neglect, confirmed
995.85	T74.01XA	Initial encounter
995.85	T74.01XD	Subsequent encounter
		Spouse or partner neglect, suspected
995.85	T76.01XA	Initial encounter
995.85	T76.01XD	Subsequent encounter
		Other circumstances related to spouse or partner neglect
V61.11	Z69.11	Encounter for mental health services for victim of spouse or partner neglect
V15.42	Z91.412	Personal history (past history) of spouse or partner neglect
V61.12	Z69.12	Encounter for mental health services for perpetrator of spouse or partner neglect
		Spouse or partner abuse, psychological, confirmed
995.82	T74.31XA	Initial encounter
995.82	T74.31XD	Subsequent encounter
		Spouse or partner abuse, psychological, suspected
995.82	T76.31XA	Initial encounter
995.82	T76.31XD	Subsequent encounter
		Other circumstances related to spouse or partner abuse, psychological
V61.11	Z69.11	Encounter for mental health services for victim of spouse or partner psychological abuse

ICD-9-CM code	ICD-10-CM code	Description
		Other circumstances related to spouse or partner abuse, psychological *(continued)*
V15.42	Z91.411	Personal history (past history) of spouse or partner psychological abuse
V61.12	Z69.12	Encounter for mental health services for perpetrator of spouse or partner psychological abuse
		Adult physical abuse by nonspouse or nonpartner, confirmed
995.81	T74.11XA	Initial encounter
995.81	T74.11XD	Subsequent encounter
		Adult physical abuse by nonspouse or nonpartner, suspected
995.81	T76.11XA	Initial encounter
995.81	T76.11XD	Subsequent encounter
		Adult sexual abuse by nonspouse or nonpartner, confirmed
995.83	T74.21XA	Initial encounter
995.83	T74.21XD	Subsequent encounter
		Adult sexual abuse by nonspouse or nonpartner, suspected
995.83	T76.21XA	Initial encounter
995.83	T76.21XD	Subsequent encounter
		Adult psychological abuse by nonspouse or nonpartner, confirmed
995.82	T74.31XA	Initial encounter
995.82	T74.31XD	Subsequent encounter

ICD-9-CM code	ICD-10-CM code	Description
		Adult psychological abuse by nonspouse or nonpartner, suspected
995.82	T76.31XA	Initial encounter
995.82	T76.31XD	Subsequent encounter
		Other circumstances related to adult abuse by nonspouse or nonpartner
V65.49	Z69.81	Encounter for mental health services for victim of nonspousal adult abuse
V62.83	Z69.82	Encounter for mental health services for perpetrator of nonspousal adult abuse
V62.3	Z55.9	Academic or educational problem
V62.21	Z56.82	Problem related to current military deployment status
V62.29	Z56.9	Other problem related to employment
V60.0	Z59.0	Homelessness
V60.1	Z59.1	Inadequate housing
V60.89	Z59.2	Discord with neighbor, lodger, or landlord
V60.6	Z59.3	Problem related to living in a residential institution
V60.2	Z59.4	Lack of adequate food or safe drinking water
V60.2	Z59.5	Extreme poverty
V60.2	Z59.6	Low income
V60.2	Z59.7	Insufficient social insurance or welfare support
V60.9	Z59.9	Unspecified housing or economic problem
V62.89	Z60.0	Phase of life problem
V60.3	Z60.2	Problem related to living alone

ICD-9-CM code	ICD-10-CM code	Description
V62.4	Z60.3	Acculturation difficulty
V62.4	Z60.4	Social exclusion or rejection
V62.4	Z60.5	Target of (perceived) adverse discrimination or persecution
V62.9	Z60.9	Unspecified problem related to social environment
V62.89	Z65.4	Victim of crime
V62.5	Z65.0	Conviction in civil or criminal proceedings without imprisonment
V62.5	Z65.1	Imprisonment or other incarceration
V62.5	Z65.2	Problems related to release from prison
V62.5	Z65.3	Problems related to other legal circumstances
V65.49	Z70.9	Sex counseling
V65.40	Z71.9	Other counseling or consultation
V62.89	Z65.8	Religious or spiritual problem
V61.7	Z64.0	Problems related to unwanted pregnancy
V61.5	Z64.1	Problems related to multiparity
V62.89	Z64.4	Discord with social service provider, including probation officer, case manager, or social services worker
V62.89	Z65.4	Victim of terrorism or torture

ICD-9-CM code	ICD-10-CM code	Description
V62.22	Z65.5	Exposure to disaster, war, or other hostilities
V62.89	Z65.8	Other problem related to psychosocial circumstances
V62.9	Z65.9	Unspecified problem related to unspecified psychosocial circumstances
V15.49	Z91.49	Other personal history of psychological trauma
V15.59	Z91.5	Personal history of self-harm
V62.22	Z91.82	Personal history of military deployment
V15.89	Z91.89	Other personal risk factors
V69.9	Z72.9	Problem related to lifestyle
V71.01	Z72.811	Adult antisocial behavior
V71.02	Z72.810	Child or adolescent antisocial behavior
V63.9	Z75.3	Unavailability or inaccessibility of health care facilities
V63.8	Z75.4	Unavailability or inaccessibility of other helping agencies
V15.81	Z91.19	Nonadherence to medical treatment
278.00	E66.9	Overweight or obesity
V65.2	Z76.5	Malingering
V40.31	Z91.83	Wandering associated with a mental disorder
V62.89	R41.83	Borderline intellectual functioning

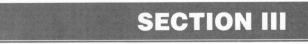

SECTION III

Chapter 7

A Brief Version of DSM-5

Diagnosis	Criteria/time	Symptoms
Neurodevelopmental disorders		
Autism spectrum disorder	All 3 beginning in early childhood *AND*	Deficits in social-emotional reciprocity; deficits in nonverbal communicative behaviors; deficits in developing and maintaining relationships
	≥2	Stereotyped or repetitive speech, motor movements, or use of objects; excessive adherence to routines or excessive resistance to change; highly restricted, fixated interests of abnormal intensity or focus; hyperreactivity or hyporeactivity to sensory input
Attention-deficit/ hyperactivity disorder	≥6 for ≥6 months *OR*	Inattention: makes careless mistakes; cannot sustain attention; does not seem to listen; often does not follow through; struggles to organize tasks; dislikes mental effort; loses objects necessary for tasks; distractible; forgetful
	≥6 for ≥6 months	Hyperactivity/impulsivity: fidgets; leaves seat; runs or climbs; unable to remain quiet; on the go; talks excessively; blurts out answers; cannot wait turn; interrupts; acts without thinking

The Pocket Guide to the DSM-5 Diagnostic Exam

Diagnosis	Criteria/time	Symptoms
Schizophrenia spectrum and other psychotic disorders		
Schizophrenia	≥2 for ≥1 month *AND*	Delusions; hallucinations; disorganized speech; grossly disorganized or catatonic behavior; negative symptoms (at least one symptom must be delusions, hallucinations, or disorganized speech)
	≥6 months	Continuous signs of disturbance
Schizoaffective disorder		Criteria for schizophrenia
	≥50% of the time *AND*	Also experiences major depressive or manic episodes
	≥2 weeks	Delusions or hallucinations without depressive or manic episodes
Bipolar and related disorders		
Bipolar I disorder	≥3 for ≥1 week (or any duration if hospitalized)	Mania: inflated self-esteem or grandiosity; decreased need for sleep; pressured speech; racing thoughts; distractibility; increased goal-directed activity; risky behavior
Bipolar II disorder	≥3 for ≥4 days	Hypomania: inflated self-esteem or grandiosity; decreased need for sleep; pressured speech; racing thoughts; distractibility; increased goal-directed activity; risky behavior *without* psychosis or hospitalization

Diagnosis	Criteria/time	Symptoms
Depressive disorders		
Major depressive disorder	≥1 for ≥2 weeks *AND*	Depressed mood; lost of interest in activities or pleasure (anhedonia)
	≥4 for ≥2 weeks	Weight loss or decreased appetite; insomnia/hypersomnia; agitation/retardation; fatigue or loss of energy; excessive guilt; decreased ability to concentrate; thoughts of death or suicide
Anxiety disorders		
Panic disorder	≥4 *AND*	Palpitations; sweating; trembling; shortness of breath; choking; chest pain; nausea; dizziness; chills; paresthesias; derealization; fear of insanity; fear of death
	≥1 month	Persistent concern or worry *OR* Maladaptive change in behavior related to attack
Generalized anxiety disorder	≥3 for ≥6 months	Restlessness; easy fatigability; difficulty concentrating; irritability; muscle tension; sleep disturbance; avoidance of situations

Diagnosis	Criteria/time	Symptoms
Obsessive-compulsive and related disorders		
Obsessive-compulsive disorder	≥1 hour/day	Obsessions: recurrent and intrusive thoughts, urges, and images that a person attempts to ignore or suppress through compulsive acts *AND/OR* Compulsions: repetitive behaviors or mental acts to reduce distress
Trauma- and stressor-related disorders		
Posttraumatic stress disorder		Exposure to trauma
	≥1 for ≥1 month *AND*	Intrusions: memories; dreams; flashbacks; exposure distress; physiological reactions
	≥1 for ≥1 month	Avoidance: internal reminders; external reminders
	≥2 for ≥1 month *AND*	Negative symptoms: impaired memory of trauma; negative self-worth; pathological blame; negative emotions; decreased participation; detachment; emotional numbness
	≥2 for ≥1 month	Arousal: irritability or aggression; recklessness; hypervigilance; exaggerated startle; impaired concentration; sleep disturbance

Diagnosis	Criteria/time	Symptoms
Neurocognitive disorders		
Delirium	Acute	Disturbance of consciousness; acute change from baseline, generally with fluctuating severity; cognitive change
Major neurocognitive disorder	Insidious	Significant cognitive decline, ≥2 SDs below normal, which interferes with independence
Mild neurocognitive disorder	Insidious	Minor cognitive decline, 1–2 SDs below normal, which does not interfere with independence (but greater effort, compensatory strategies, or accommodations may be required)

Chapter 8

A Stepwise Approach to Differential Diagnosis

Although diagnoses are the stated product of a diagnostic interview, a good diagnostic interviewer should generate more hypotheses than diagnoses, because an interviewer is investigating the nature of a person's distress (Feinstein 1967). In these investigations, you should consider a diverse set of possibilities. Although several manuals have been designed specifically to teach the differential diagnosis for DSM-5 (Barnhill 2014; Black and Grant 2014; First 2014; Roberts and Louie 2014), it is helpful to review the following general six-step approach to generating the differential diagnosis. As you develop your clinical decision making, it is helpful to follow these steps sequentially so you develop the habit of considering what Kenneth Kendler (2012, p. 377) calls "the dappled nature," the many and interrelated causes, of mental disorders.

Step 1: Consider to What Extent the Signs and Symptoms Are Intentionally Produced

Always consider if a patient is intentionally producing findings. If intentionally produced findings are associated with an obvious external award—such as money, disability, or time off—consider the possibility of malingering. Remember that malingering can be concomitant with other medical and psychiatric diagnoses.

If intentionally produced findings are associated with the desire to be perceived as ill or impaired, consider factitious disorder.

A patient can also unconsciously produce signs or symptoms to resolve a conflict, to validate his inability to function, or as an attempt to secure assistance. In these situations, consider a somatic disorder.

Step 2: Consider to What Extent the Signs and Symptoms Are Related to Substances

The variety of substances that people use and misuse is remarkable, as are the clinical effects of substance use. People can experience mental distress during substance use, intoxication, and withdrawal. When you seek the cause of a patient's distress, always consider drugs of abuse, as well as prescription, over-the-counter, and herbal medicines. People often underreport their use of substances, so consider these possibilities:

- Substances directly cause his psychiatric signs and symptoms.
- A patient uses substances because of a mental disorder and its sequelae.
- A patient uses substances and experiences psychiatric signs and symptoms, but the substance use and the signs/symptoms are unrelated.

Step 3: Consider to What Extent the Signs and Symptoms Are Related to Another Medical Condition

A patient can present with another medical condition that mimics psychiatric signs and symptoms. Sometimes, his presentation with these findings is a sentinel event that occurs in advance of the other stigmata of a medical condition. Alternatively, he may develop psychiatric signs and symptoms years after his presentation for another medical condition. Clues that another medical condition may be related to a mental disorder include an atypical presentation, abnormal age at onset, and abnormal course. Consider these possibilities:

- Another medical condition directly alters his psychiatric signs and symptoms.
- Another medical condition indirectly alters his psychiatric signs and symptoms, as through a psychological mechanism.
- The treatment for another medical condition directly alters his psychiatric signs and symptoms.

- His mental disorder, or its treatment, causes or exacerbates another medical condition.
- A patient has a mental disorder and another medical condition, but they are causally unrelated.

Step 4: Consider to What Extent the Signs and Symptoms Are Related to a Developmental Conflict or Stage

If you are evaluating a young child, your diagnostic interview should include formal developmental testing, a skill beyond the scope of this book. Even when you are interviewing older children, adolescents, and adults, however, you should consider a patient's developmental stage, which can be quite different from the developmental stage you would expect based on his age, background, and education. A thorough social history will give you a sense of how his current behavior relates to his usual behavior, but it is also useful to observe how your patient communicates and behaves, and compare his communication and behavior with those appropriate for his age. If you observe a disjunction in any patients, consider these possibilities:

- They are experiencing a transient regression in response to a particular event.
- They are employing an immature defense mechanism, which may indicate a personality trait or disorder.
- They are experiencing a developmental conflict in a particular relationship.
- They have a developmental delay.

Step 5: Consider to What Extent the Signs and Symptoms Are Related to a Mental Disorder

"Normality" covers a wide range of behaviors and thoughts that vary across cultural groups and developmental stages. In DSM-5, a mental disturbance must cause "clinically significant disturbance in an individual's cognition, emotion regulation, or behavior that reflects a dysfunction in the psychological, biological, or developmental processes underlying mental functioning" (American Psychiatric Association 2013, p. 20) to be considered a disorder rather than just a constellation of symptoms. Diagnoses are summaries of information that allow you to categorize the experiences of a distressed person and to communicate with his other professionals, and you should rely on the predominant symptomatology to support your diagnosis. DSM-5 seeks parsimony, but diagnoses are not mutually exclusive, so consider these possibilities:

- Condition A predisposes a patient to Condition B, and vice versa.
- An underlying condition, such as a genetic predisposition, may predispose a patient to both Conditions A and B.
- A mediating factor, such as alterations in reward systems, may influence a patient's susceptibility to both Conditions A and B.
- Conditions A and B may be part of a more complex and unified syndrome that has been artificially split in the diagnostic system.
- The relationship between Conditions A and B may be artificially enhanced by overlaps in the diagnostic criteria.
- The comorbidity between Conditions A and B may be coincidental.

Step 6: Consider Whether No Mental Disorder Is Present

When a patient's symptoms and presentation do not fulfill the criteria for a specific mental disorder but cause clinically significant distress or impairment, consider alternatives. If the distress or impairment has developed as a maladaptive response to an identifiable psychosocial stressor, consider an adjustment disorder. If the patient's symptoms are not secondary to a stressor, consider an other specified or unspecified diagnosis, or the possibility he has no psychiatric diagnosis at all.

Chapter 9

The Mental Status Examination: A Psychiatric Glossary

Just as a physical examination commonly moves from head to toe, the mental status examination begins with a person's outer appearances and progressively proceeds into her interior life. To describe these experiences, clinicians use a specialized language. Comprehensive glossaries of psychiatric terms are available elsewhere (see Shahrokh et al. 2011 and the appendix to DSM-5). The following list includes both brief definitions of some of the more specialized terms used in the mental status examination and a way to organize your findings.

Mental Status Examination

Appearance

Note a person's dress, cleanliness, habitus, posture, appropriateness for her age, and ability to form and maintain eye contact.

Behavior

Describe any mannerisms (peculiar and characteristic goal-directed behaviors), stereotypies (repetitive and abnormal non-goal-directed behavior), posturing (striking a pose and maintaining it), presence of waxy flexibility (resistance of limbs to passive motion), catalepsy (maintaining of any position), tremor, agitation, psychomotor retardation, or signs of extrapyramidal symptoms or tardive dyskinesia.

Speech

Describe the rate, tone, rhythm, volume, general quality, and presence of any latency (a pause of several seconds before responding to a question).

Emotion

Describe the quality, type, stability, range, intensity, and appropriateness of a person's emotional state. Describe the person's mood, sustained emotional state, and affect (i.e., the observable behaviors that are expressions of emotion).

Thought Process

Describe how a person thinks, and note any evidence of loosening of her associations—ranging from intact, circumstantial (providing unnecessary details but eventually answering a question), tangential (only touching upon the question at hand), loose (providing responses unrelated to a question), and flight of ideas (nearly continuous flow of speech based on an understandable but distracting group of associations) to word salad (random use of words). Also observe for distractibility (being easily diverted by extraneous stimuli), derailment (running ideas into each other), perseveration, verbigeration (prolonged repetition of isolated words), echolalia (repetition of words or statements of others), neologisms (creation of words), clang association (choosing words purely for sound), alliteration, push of speech (increased, rapid speech that is often loud and difficult to interrupt), decreased latency of response (answering questions before you can finish asking them), increased latency of response, poverty of speech, blocking (sudden stops in the middle of a thought sequence), mutism (absence of speech), and aphonia (ability to only whisper or croak).

Thought Content

Comment on what a person discusses, including the presence of ideation, intent, or plan to harm self or others; phobias (intense, unreasonable fears of a specific object, activity, or situation); obsession (recurrent, persistent idea, image, or desire that dominates thought); compulsion (irresistible impulse to perform an action); hallucination (the perception of an absent stimulus); illusion (misperception of an actual stimulus); delusions (fixed, firm, false beliefs that are not part of a person's culture or religion); persecution; paranoia; grandiosity; thought insertion; thought withdrawal; guilt; passivity; and ideas of reference (perceptions that unrelated stimuli have a particular and unusual meaning specific to the person).

Cognition and Intellectual Resources

Observe a person's orientation, recent and remote memory, ability to calculate, and ability to abstract and to interpret proverbs. Comment on the person's insight and judgment, especially as they relate to the presenting condition.

Chapter 10

The American Board of Psychiatry and Neurology Clinical Skills Evaluation

If you are a psychiatrist seeking board certification, you must first demonstrate your ability to interview and present a patient, whom you have never previously met, while being directly observed by a board-certified psychiatrist. The patient must be an actual rather than a standardized patient. Although each residency training program has its own set of rules for observing these interviews, called *clinical skills evaluations,* the American Board of Psychiatry and Neurology (ABPN) has established requirements for qualifying interviews.

The ABPN requires that an applicant pass three of these evaluations with three separate patients. Each evaluation must include at least 30 minutes to interview a patient and an additional 15 minutes to present the case, but resident training programs can provide additional time at their discretion. The evaluations can occur at any point in a resident's training. Regardless of when a trainee is examined, the trainee must perform the interview at a level consistent with that of a currently practicing psychiatrist to pass an evaluation.

Faculty members evaluate an applicant's ability to perform three skills: form a patient-physician relationship, obtain a psychiatric history, and present a case. Faculty members are asked to rate a resident's ability to perform each skill and to rate constituent skills, on a scale from 1 to 8, with scores from 1 to 4 being unacceptable and scores from 5 to 8 being acceptable. For an examinee to pass the examination, a faculty member must score the resident at 5 or above on each skill.

Before taking the examination, you should familiarize yourself with the evaluation form that will be used. The ABPN makes the form freely available on its Web site (www.abpn.com/psych.html), along with additional details about board certification.

I provide advice on how to interview and present a patient in Chapter 3, "The 30-Minute Diagnostic Interview." Remember that your goal is to show how you relate to and understand a person presenting with mental distress, and keep in mind that the most important skill to demonstrate is your ability to form a therapeutic alliance.

Chapter 11

Selected DSM-5 Assessment Measures

In addition to its categorical diagnoses, DSM-5 includes a number of cross-cutting symptom and other assessment measures. These measures are useful for screening for mental disorders, for characterizing the degree of functional impairment associated with a mental disorder, and for prioritizing a particular area of clinical concern. Because I designed this book for the diagnostic interview, I include in this chapter only the tools that will be most useful for the diagnostic interview. The full range of assessment measures relevant to DSM-5, including those for diagnostic severity, can be found online at www.psychiatry.org/dsm5.

Cultural Formulation Interview

As discussed in Chapter 4 ("Adventures in Dimensions"), the Cultural Formulation Interview (CFI) is not a scored rating system, but rather a series of prompts to help you explore a person's understanding of illness and health. The CFI can be incorporated into a diagnostic examination when you want to personalize the diagnosis and build a therapeutic alliance. The complete CFI, which is in Section III of DSM-5, includes additional questions that expand upon each domain. What follows here is an operationalized adaptation divided into six themes. Just as in the rest of the book, the italicized portions are interview prompts.

Introduction: *I would like to understand the problems that bring you here so that I can help you more effectively. I want to know about your experience and ideas. I will ask some questions about what is going on and how you are dealing with it. There are no right or wrong answers. I just want to know your views and those of other important people in your life.*

Cultural definition of the problem: *What problems or concerns bring you to the clinic? What troubles you most about your problem? People often understand their problems in their own way, which may be similar to or different from how doctors explain the problem. How would you describe your problem to someone else? Sometimes people use particular words or phrases to talk about their problems. Is there a specific term or expression that describes your problem? If yes: What is it?*

Cultural perceptions of cause and context: *Why do you think this is happening to you? What do you think are the particular causes of your problem? Some people may explain their problem as the result of bad things that happen in their lives, problems with others, or a physical illness. Or they give a spiritual reason for, or identify some other cause of, their problem. Do you? What, if anything, makes your problem worse, or makes it harder to cope with? What have your family, friends, and other people in your life done that may have made your problem worse? What, if anything, makes your problem better, or helps you cope with it more easily?*

Role of cultural identity: *Is there anything about your background—for example, your culture, race, ethnicity, religion, or geographical origin—that is causing problems for you in your current life situation? If yes: In what way? On the other hand, is there anything about your background that helps you to cope with your current life situation? If yes: In what way?*

Cultural factors affecting self-coping and past help seeking: *Sometimes people consider various ways of making themselves feel better. What have you done on your own to cope with your problem? Often, people also look for help from other individuals, groups, or institutions to help them feel better. In the past, what kind of treatment or help from other sources have you sought for your problem? What type of help or treatment was most useful? How? What type of help or treatment was not useful? How? Has anything prevented you from getting the help you need—for example, cost or lack of insurance coverage, getting time off work or family responsibilities, concern about stigma or discrimination, or lack of services that understand your language or culture? If yes: What got in the way?*

Current help seeking: *Now let's talk about the help you would be getting here. Is there anything about my own background that might make it difficult for me to understand or help you with your problem? How can I and others at our facility be most helpful to you? What kind of help would you like from us now, as specialists in mental health?*

Conclusion: Thank the person for participation, summarize the main findings, and transition back to the remainder of your interview.

World Health Organization Disability Assessment Schedule 2.0

As part of their efforts to synchronize DSM with international diagnostic tools, the authors of DSM-5 have adopted the World Health Organization Disability Assessment Schedule 2.0 (WHODAS 2.0) to assess a person's function in six domains: cognition, mobility, self-care, getting along, life activities, and participation. WHODAS 2.0 is available in several versions: 12- and 36-question versions that can be self-administered, proxy administered, or interviewer administered (see World Health Organization 2010).

For the purposes of a DSM-5 diagnostic interview, DSM-5 includes the 36-item self-administered version in Section III. WHODAS 2.0 includes background questions about age, gender, educational attainment, and marital and occupational status. The WHODAS 2.0 developers recommend administering the examination using flashcards with some of this material printed on them. You can obtain these flashcards, along with other versions of WHODAS 2.0, online at www.who.int/classifications/icf/whodasii/en.

Clinician-Rated Dimensions of Psychosis Symptom Severity

The Clinician-Rated Dimensions of Psychosis Symptom Severity is an 8-item measure that may be completed by the clinician at the time of the clinical assessment. Each item asks the clinician to rate the severity of each symptom as experienced by the individual during the past 7 days.

Name: _____   Age: _____   Sex: [ ] Male   Date: _____
                                                  [ ] Female

Instructions: Based on all the information you have on the individual and using your clinical judgment, please rate (with checkmark) the presence and severity of the following symptoms as experienced by the individual in the past seven (7) days.

Domain	0	1	2	3	4	Score
I. Hallucinations	☐ Not present	☐ Equivocal (severity or duration not sufficient to be considered psychosis)	☐ Present, but mild (little pressure to act upon voices, not very bothered by voices)	☐ Present and moderate (some pressure to respond to voices, or is somewhat bothered by voices)	☐ Present and severe (severe pressure to respond to voices, or is very bothered by voices)	
II. Delusions	☐ Not present	☐ Equivocal (severity or duration not sufficient to be considered psychosis)	☐ Present, but mild (little pressure to act upon delusional beliefs, not very bothered by beliefs)	☐ Present and moderate (some pressure to act upon beliefs, or is somewhat bothered by beliefs)	☐ Present and severe (severe pressure to act upon beliefs, or is very bothered by beliefs)	
III. Disorganized speech	☐ Not present	☐ Equivocal (severity or duration not sufficient to be considered disorganization)	☐ Present, but mild (some difficulty following speech)	☐ Present and moderate (speech often difficult to follow)	☐ Present and severe (speech almost impossible to follow)	

Domain	0	1	2	3	4	Score
IV. Abnormal psychomotor behavior	☐ Not present	☐ Equivocal (severity or duration not sufficient to be considered abnormal psychomotor behavior)	☐ Present, but mild (occasional abnormal or bizarre motor behavior or catatonia)	☐ Present and moderate (frequent abnormal or bizarre motor behavior or catatonia)	☐ Present and severe (abnormal or bizarre motor behavior or catatonia almost constant)	
V. Negative symptoms (restricted emotional expression or avolition)	☐ Not present	☐ Equivocal decrease in facial expressivity, prosody, gestures, or self-initiated behavior	☐ Present, but mild decrease in facial expressivity, prosody, gestures, or self-initiated behavior	☐ Present and moderate decrease in facial expressivity, prosody, gestures, or self-initiated behavior	☐ Present and severe decrease in facial expressivity, prosody, gestures, or self-initiated behavior	
VI. Impaired cognition	☐ Not present	☐ Equivocal (cognitive function not clearly outside the range expected for age or SES; i.e., within 0.5 SD of mean)	☐ Present, but mild (some reduction in cognitive function; below expected for age and SES, 0.5–1 SD from mean)	☐ Present and moderate (clear reduction in cognitive function; below expected for age and SES, 1–2 SD from mean)	☐ Present and severe (severe reduction in cognitive function; below expected for age and SES, > 2 SD from mean)	

Selected DSM-5 Assessment Measures   **213**

Domain	0	1	2	3	4	Score
VII. Depression	☐ Not present	☐ Equivocal (occasionally feels sad, down, depressed, or hopeless; concerned about having failed someone or at something but not preoccupied)	☐ Present, but mild (frequent periods of feeling very sad, down, moderately depressed, or hopeless; concerned about having failed someone or at something, with some preoccupation)	☐ Present and moderate (frequent periods of deep depression or hopelessness; preoccupation with guilt, having done wrong)	☐ Present and severe (deeply depressed or hopeless daily; delusional guilt or unreasonable self-reproach grossly out of proportion to circumstances)	
VIII. Mania	☐ Not present	☐ Equivocal (occasional elevated, expansive, or irritable mood or some restlessness)	☐ Present, but mild (frequent periods of somewhat elevated, expansive, or irritable mood or restlessness)	☐ Present and moderate (frequent periods of extensively elevated, expansive, or irritable mood or restlessness)	☐ Present and severe (daily and extensively elevated, expansive, or irritable mood or restlessness)	

Note. SD = standard deviation; SES = socioeconomic status.

Chapter 12

Dimensional Diagnosis of Personality Disorders

DSM-5 includes two distinct methods for diagnosing personality traits and disorders. The first method is a *categorical* method familiar to interviewers accustomed to DSM-IV (and DSM-IV-TR). This categorical method is included in the main section of DSM-5 for clinical use and is incorporated into the diagnostic interview in Chapters 3 ("The 30-Minute Diagnostic Interview") and 6 ("The DSM-5 Diagnostic Interview") of this pocket guide. However, the second method is a *dimensional* method that will be novel for most interviewers. At present, the dimensional model is recommended for the use of researchers but is included in Section III of DSM-5 as an emerging model that may eventually replace the more-familiar categorical model. To prepare ourselves, I thought it helpful to introduce the dimensional model in this chapter.

The dimensional model of personality disorders requires an introduction because it initially appears clinically unwieldy. The personality disorders are organized not by outward appearances into Clusters A, B, and C, but by their underlying personality traits. So you can, for example, observe submissive traits in one patient that meet criteria for borderline personality disorder while the same traits in another patient meet the criteria for avoidant personality disorder, without diagnosing separate personality disorders. As a result, several of the personality disorders in the categorical model are not included in the dimensional model. The dimensional model also allows you to go beyond determining if a person does (or does not) have a personality disorder, to assess the extent to which a personality disorder is associated with functional impairment in her relationships with other people and her sense of self. In short, if the disadvantage of the dimensional model is our lack of familiarity, its advantage is that it allows us to produce more sophisticated accounts of a person's character structure.

In this chapter, I include three tools to introduce the dimensional model of personality disorders. The first, the Level of Personality Functioning Scale, is also found in Section III of DSM-5. The scale allows you to assess the level of functional impairment associated with the personality traits or disorders you diagnose. The second, the Personality Trait Rating Form, is also found in Section III of DSM-5. This form allows you to observe the presence and severity of the 25 traits that underlie personality disorders. The third, a diagnostic interview, draws on the proposed dimensional diagnostic criteria for personality disorders in Section III of DSM-5. As in the other sections of this pocket guide, it begins with a screening question and is followed by subsequent questions to determine a specific diagnosis.

Level of Personality Functioning Scale

For each person you evaluate, DSM-5 advises evaluation of his personality traits in relation to his ability to function both personally and interpersonally. This evaluation can guide treatment planning and influence prognosis, as discussed in Chapter 4, "Adventures in Dimensions."

In order to use it, you need sufficient clinical and historical information to differentiate five levels of functioning impairment, ranging from *little or no impairment* (Level 0) to *extreme impairment* (Level 4).

Using the following descriptions as your guide, indicate the level that most closely characterizes a patient's self-functioning and interpersonal functioning.

	Self		Interpersonal	
Level	Identity	Self-Direction	Empathy	Intimacy
0 (Little or no impairment)	• Ongoing awareness of a unique self; maintains role-appropriate boundaries. • Consistent and self-regulated positive self-esteem, with accurate self-appraisal. • Capable of experiencing, tolerating, and regulating a full range of emotions.	• Sets and aspires to reasonable goals based on a realistic assessment of personal capacities. • Utilizes appropriate standards of behavior, attaining fulfillment in multiple realms. • Can reflect on, and make constructive meaning of, internal experience.	• Capable of accurately understanding others' experiences and motivations in most situations. • Comprehends and appreciates others' perspectives, even if disagreeing. • Is aware of the effect of own actions on others.	• Maintains multiple satisfying and enduring relationships in personal and community life. • Desires and engages in a number of caring, close, and reciprocal relationships. • Strives for cooperation and mutual benefit and flexibly responds to a range of others' ideas, emotions, and behaviors.

Level	Self		Interpersonal	
	Identity	Self-Direction	Empathy	Intimacy
1 (Some impairment)	• Relatively intact sense of self, with some decrease in clarity of boundaries when strong emotions and mental distress are experienced. • Self-esteem diminished at times, with overly critical or somewhat distorted self-appraisal. • Strong emotions may be distressing, associated with a restriction in range of emotional experience.	• Excessively goal-directed, somewhat goal-inhibited, or conflicted about goals. • May have an unrealistic or socially inappropriate set of personal standards, limiting some aspects of fulfillment. • Able to reflect on internal experiences, but may overemphasize a single (e.g., intellectual, emotional) type of self-knowledge.	• Somewhat compromised in ability to appreciate and understand others' experiences; may tend to see others as having unreasonable expectations or a wish for control. • Although capable of considering and understanding different perspectives, resists doing so. • Inconsistent in awareness of effect of own behavior on others.	• Able to establish enduring relationships in personal and community life, with some limitations on degree of depth and satisfaction. • Capacity and desire to form intimate and reciprocal relationships, but may be inhibited in meaningful expression and sometimes constrained if intense emotions or conflicts arise. • Cooperation may be inhibited by unrealistic standards; somewhat limited in ability to respect or respond to others' ideas, emotions, and behaviors.

Level	Self		Interpersonal	
	Identity	Self-Direction	Empathy	Intimacy
2 (Moderate impairment)	• Excessive dependence on others for identity definition, with compromised boundary delineation. • Vulnerable self-esteem controlled by exaggerated concern about external evaluation, with a wish for approval. Sense of incompleteness or inferiority, with compensatory inflated, or deflated, self-appraisal. • Emotional regulation depends on positive external appraisal. Threats to self-esteem may engender strong emotions such as rage or shame.	• Goals are more often a means of gaining external approval than self-generated, and thus may lack coherence and/or stability. • Personal standards may be unreasonably high (e.g., a need to be special or please others) or low (e.g., not consonant with prevailing social values). Fulfillment is compromised by a sense of lack of authenticity. • Impaired capacity to reflect upon internal experience.	• Hyperattuned to the experience of others, but only with respect to perceived relevance to self. • Excessively self-referential; significantly compromised ability to appreciate and understand others' experiences and to consider alternative perspectives. • Generally unaware of or unconcerned about effect of own behavior on others, or unrealistic appraisal of own effect.	• Capacity and desire to form relationships in personal and community life, but connections may be largely superficial. • Intimate relationships are largely based on meeting self-regulatory and self-esteem needs, with an unrealistic expectation of being perfectly understood by others. • Tends not to view relationships in reciprocal terms, and cooperates predominantly for personal gain.

	Self			Interpersonal	
Level	Identity	Self-Direction	Empathy	Intimacy	
3 (Severe impairment)	• A weak sense of autonomy/ agency; experience of a lack of identity, or emptiness. Boundary definition is poor or rigid: may be overidentification with others, overemphasis on independence from others, or vacillation between these.	• Difficulty establishing and/or achieving personal goals.	• Ability to consider and understand the thoughts, feelings, and behavior of other people is significantly limited; may discern very specific aspects of others' experience, particularly vulnerabilities and suffering.	• Some desire to form relationships in community and personal life is present, but capacity for positive and enduring connection is significantly impaired.	
		• Internal standards for behavior are unclear or contradictory. Life is experienced as meaningless or dangerous.			
	• Fragile self-esteem is easily influenced by events, and self-image lacks coherence. Self-appraisal is unnuanced: self-loathing, self-aggrandizing, or an illogical, unrealistic combination.	• Significantly compromised ability to reflect upon and understand own mental processes.	• Generally unable to consider alternative perspectives; highly threatened by differences of opinion or alternative viewpoints.	• Relationships are based on a strong belief in the absolute need for the intimate other(s), and/or expectations of abandonment or abuse. Feelings about intimate involvement with others alternate between fear/rejection and desperate desire for connection.	
	• Emotions may be rapidly shifting or a chronic, unwavering feeling of despair.		• Confusion or unawareness of impact of own actions on others; often bewildered about peoples' thoughts and actions, with destructive motivations frequently misattributed to others.	• Little mutuality: others are conceptualized primarily in terms of how they affect the self (negatively or positively); cooperative efforts are often disrupted due to the perception of slights from others.	

Level	Self		Interpersonal	
	Identity	Self-Direction	Empathy	Intimacy
4 (Extreme impairment)	• Experience of a unique self and sense of agency/autonomy are virtually absent, or are organized around perceived external persecution. Boundaries with others are confused or lacking. • Weak or distorted self-image easily threatened by interactions with others; significant distortions and confusion around self-appraisal. Emotions not congruent with context or internal experience. Hatred and aggression may be dominant affects, although they may be disavowed and attributed to others.	• Poor differentiation of thoughts from actions, so goal-setting ability is severely compromised, with unrealistic or incoherent goals. • Internal standards for behavior are virtually lacking. Genuine fulfillment is virtually inconceivable. • Profound inability to constructively reflect upon own experience. Personal motivations may be unrecognized and/or experienced as external to self.	• Pronounced inability to consider and understand others' experience and motivation. • Attention to others' perspectives virtually absent (attention is hypervigilant, focused on need fulfillment and harm avoidance). • Social interactions can be confusing and disorienting.	• Desire for affiliation is limited because of profound disinterest or expectation of harm. Engagement with others is detached, disorganized, or consistently negative. • Relationships are conceptualized almost exclusively in terms of their ability to provide comfort or inflict pain and suffering. Social/interpersonal behavior is not reciprocal; rather, it seeks fulfillment of basic needs or escape from pain.

Personality Trait Rating Form

As discussed in Chapters 5 ("Key Changes in DSM-5") and 6, it is sometimes clinically useful to create a detailed portrait of a person's personality traits. In the dimensional DSM-5 model for personality disorders, this is done by rating domains and facets of a person's usual personality—what they have been for the majority of the person's adult life. For each domain and facet, you rate how well the description assesses the person before you on this 4-point scale:

0	1	2	3
Very little or not at all descriptive	Mildly descriptive	Moderately descriptive	Extremely descriptive

Rating	Negative affectivity	Experiences negative emotions frequently and intensely

NOTE: Restricted Affectivity is listed under the Detachment heading, but the absence of this facet trait—i.e., a tendency to have strong reactions to emotionally arousing situations, should also be evaluated in rating the overall Negative Affectivity domain.

Emotional lability	Unstable emotional experiences and frequent mood changes; emotions that are easily aroused, intense, and/or out of proportion to events and circumstances
Anxiousness	Intense feelings of nervousness, tenseness, or panic in reaction to diverse situations; worry about the negative effects of past unpleasant experiences and future negative possibilities; feeling fearful, apprehensive, or threatened by uncertainty; fears of falling apart, losing control, or embarrassment
Separation insecurity	Fears of rejection by—and/or separation from—significant others, associated with fears of excessive dependency and complete loss of autonomy
Perseveration	Persistence at tasks long after the behavior has ceased to be functional or effective; continuance of the same behavior despite repeated failures
Submissiveness	Adaptation of one's behavior to the interests and desires of others
Hostility	Persistent or frequent angry feelings; anger or irritability in response to minor slights and insults; mean, nasty, or vengeful behavior
Depressivity	Frequent feelings of being down, miserable, and/or hopeless; difficulty recovering from such moods; pessimism about the future; pervasive shame; feelings of inferior self-worth; thoughts of suicide and suicidal behavior
Suspiciousness	Expectations of—and heightened sensitivity to—signs of interpersonal ill-intent or harm; doubts about loyalty and fidelity of others; feelings of persecution

Rating	Detachment	Withdrawal from other people and from social interactions

NOTE: Because they are rated earlier, as part of Negative Affectivity, Depressivity and Suspiciousness are not listed again under the Detachment heading, but they should be evaluated in rating the overall Detachment domain.

	Restricted affectivity	Little reaction to emotionally arousing situations; constricted emotional experience and expression; indifference or coldness
	Withdrawal	Preference for being alone to being with others; reticence in social situations; avoidance of social contacts and activity; lack of initiation of social contact
	Anhedonia	Lack of enjoyment from, engagement in, or energy for life's experiences; deficits in the capacity to feel pleasure or take interest in things
	Intimacy avoidance	Avoidance of close or romantic relationships, interpersonal attachments, and intimate sexual relationships

Rating	Antagonism	Engaging in behaviors that put the person at odds with other people

NOTE: Because it is rated earlier, as part of Negative Affectivity, Hostility is not listed again under the Antagonism heading, but it should be evaluated in rating the overall Antagonism domain.

	Manipulativeness	Frequent use of subterfuge to influence or control others; use of seduction, charm, glibness, or ingratiation to achieve one's ends
	Deceitfulness	Dishonesty and fraudulence; misrepresentation of self; embellishment or fabrication when relating events
	Grandiosity	Feelings of entitlement, either overt or covert; self-centeredness; firmly holding to the belief that one is better than others; condescending toward others
	Attention seeking	Excessive attempts to attract and be the focus of the attention of others; admiration seeking
	Callousness	Lack of concern for feelings or problems of others; lack of guilt or remorse about the negative or harmful effects of one's actions on others; aggression; sadism

Rating	Disinhibition/ compulsivity	Engaging in behaviors on impulse, without reflecting on potential future consequences

NOTE: Compulsivity is the opposite of disinhibition and, if present, should be recorded at the facet level as Rigid Perfectionism in the absence of other disinhibition facets. Rigid Perfectionism reflects Compulsivity, which is the opposite of disinhibition and is therefore located in the Disinhibition domain. If present, Compulsivity should be recorded at the facet level as a higher Rigid Perfectionism score accompanied by lower scores on other disinhibition facets.

Irresponsibility	Disregard for—and failure to honor—financial and other obligations or commitments; lack of respect for—and lack of follow-through on—agreements and promises
Impulsivity	Acting on the spur of the moment in response to immediate stimuli; acting on a momentary basis without a plan or consideration of outcomes; difficulty establishing and following plans; a sense of urgency and self-harming behavior under emotional distress
Distractibility	Difficulty concentrating and focusing on tasks; attention is easily diverted by extraneous stimuli; difficulty maintaining goal-focused behavior
Risk taking	Engagement in dangerous, risky, and potentially self-damaging activities, unnecessarily and without regard to consequences; boredom proneness and thoughtless initiation of activities to counter boredom; lack of concern for one's limitations and denial of the reality of personal danger
(lack of) Rigid perfectionism	Rigid insistence on everything being flawless, perfect, without errors or faults, including one's own and others' performance; sacrificing of timeliness to ensure correctness in every detail; believing that there is only one right way to do things; difficulty changing ideas and/or viewpoint; preoccupation with details, organization, and order

Rating	Psychoticism	Unusual and bizarre experiences
	Unusual beliefs and experiences	Thought content that is viewed by others as bizarre or idiosyncratic; unusual experiences of reality
	Eccentricity	Odd, unusual, or bizarre behavior or appearance; saying unusual or inappropriate things
	Cognitive and perceptual dysregulation	Odd or unusual thought processes; vague, circumstantial, metaphorical, over-elaborate, or stereotyped thought or speech; odd experiences in various sensory modalities

Screening questions: *When you look over your life, does it seem like your basic sense of who you are, your ability to accurately estimate the quality of your own life, and your ability to experience and regulate emotions have been unstable or have changed frequently? When you look over your life, does it seem like you struggled to consistently and purposefully pursue both short- and long-term goals for yourself?*

If yes to either question, ask: *When you look over your life, does it seem like you repeatedly struggle to appreciate the experiences of other people, to tolerate different perspectives, and to understand the effect of your behavior on other people? Do you really struggle to make and maintain deep positive connections with other people?*

If yes to either question, ask: *When people look over their lives, they can often identify persistent habits or traits that recur throughout their lives. When you look over your life, can you see that one of these traits is relatively stable over time: having a negative sense of yourself that changes quickly in response to circumstances; a compulsive focus on getting things perfect or rightly ordered; avoiding or withdrawing from emotional intimate relationships to the extent that you feel detached from other people; a commitment to behaviors and beliefs that many other people consider unusual or eccentric; a persistent sense that you are much more accomplished or deserving than other people; or a pattern of behaviors that many other people have found manipulative, deceitful, hostile, or irresponsible?*

- If negative affectivity as characterized by an unstable negative mood predominates, proceed to borderline personality disorder criteria.
- If compulsivity predominates, proceed to obsessive-compulsive personality disorder criteria.
- If detachment predominates, proceed to avoidant personality disorder criteria.
- If psychoticism characterized by unusual or eccentric behaviors predominate, proceed to schizotypal personality disorder criteria.
- If antagonism characterized by manipulativeness, deceitfulness, hostility and irresponsibility predominates, proceed to antisocial (dissocial) personality disorder criteria.
- If antagonism characterized by grandiosity and attention seeking predominates, proceed to narcissistic personality disorder criteria.

1. Borderline Personality Disorder

   a. Inclusion: Requires impairments in self-functioning as manifested by at least <u>one</u> of the following difficulties.

      i. Identity: *Do you have a very unstable or poorly developed sense of who you are? Are you excessively critical of yourself? Do you chronically feel empty? At times of stress, do you ever feel like you are an outside observer of your mind, thoughts, feelings, sensations, body, or your whole self or experience people or places as unreal, dreamlike, foggy, lifeless, or visually distorted?*

      ii. Self-direction: *Are your aspirations, career plans, goals, and values unstable and frequently changing?*

   b. Inclusion: Also requires impairment in interpersonal functioning as manifested by at least <u>one</u> of the following difficulties.

      i. Empathy: *Do you struggle to recognize the needs and feelings of other people? Are you prone to feeling slighted or insulted? When you think about other people, do you think mostly about their negative qualities or their weaknesses?*

      ii. Intimacy: *Do you worry that if people get close to you, they will abandon you? Are most of your close relationships intense and unstable? Do you alternate between feeling as though the people in your life are really good and really bad? Do you alternate between being really involved with other people and then withdrawing from relationships?*

   c. Inclusion: Also requires pathological personality traits from at least <u>one</u> of the following domains.

      i. Negative affectivity, characterized by at least <u>one</u> of the following:

         • Emotional lability: *Are your emotions easily aroused or intense? Are your emotions often much stronger than the event or circumstance that triggered them?*

         • Anxiousness: *Do you often have intense feelings of nervousness, tension, or panic, especially when stressed? Do you often feel afraid of uncertainty? Do you worry about how negative experiences in your past will affect your future? Do you fear falling apart or losing control?*

- Separation insecurity: *Do you really fear rejection by or separation from the people closest to you?*
- Depressivity: *Do you frequently feel down, miserable, or hopeless? Do you find it hard to recover from these moods? Are you very pessimistic about the future? Do you often feel ashamed of yourself or feel that you are worthless? Do you frequently think about harming or killing yourself?*

ii. Disinhibition, characterized by at least <u>one</u> of the following:

- Impulsivity: *Do you often act on the spur of the moment, without a plan or consideration for the outcome? Do you have difficulty establishing or following plans? When you are stressed, do you feel a sense of urgency or a desire to harm yourself?*
- Risk taking: *Do you frequently engage in dangerous, risky, and potentially self-damaging activities without regard to their consequences?*

iii. Antagonism, characterized by the following:

- Hostility: *Are you frequently angry or irritable, especially in response to minor slights and insults?*

d. Exclusions

i. If the impairments in personality functioning and the expression of personality traits are unstable over time and inconsistent across situations, do not make the diagnosis.

ii. If the impairments in personality functioning and the personality trait expressions are normative for a person's developmental stage or sociocultural environment, do not make the diagnosis.

iii. If the impairments in personality functioning and the personality trait expressions are solely associated with the direct physiological effects of another medical condition or a substance, do not make the diagnosis.

e. Modifiers

i. Descriptive features

- More pervasive negative affectivity
- More pervasive detachment
- More pervasive antagonism

- More pervasive disinhibition
- More pervasive psychoticism
- Level of personality functioning (0–4) (see Level of Personality Functioning Scale in this chapter)

    ii. Course

- In remission

  f. Alternative: If a person exhibits significant impairment in self and interpersonal functioning but does not meet criteria for a specific personality disorder, consider personality disorder—trait specified (full proposed criteria are in DSM-5, p. 770). This diagnosis allows you to specify the domains in which pathological personality domains—negative affectivity, detachment, antagonism, disinhibition, and psychoticism—are present and to diagnose the disorder. If you desire, you can use the specific trait facets within each domain to particularize the diagnosis. (You can see a list of these facets in the Personality Trait Rating Form on p. 222 of this chapter.)

2. Obsessive-Compulsive Personality Disorder

  a. Inclusion: Requires impairments in self-functioning as manifested by at least <u>one</u> of the following difficulties.

    i. Identity: *Do you find that your sense of who you are and what makes you valuable as a person comes mostly from your work or how productive you are? Is it so difficult for you to experience and express strong emotions that it would be fair to characterize your ability to do so as constricted?*

    ii. Self-direction: *Do you have such a strong need to do your work or duty well and thoroughly that you find it difficult to complete tasks? Do you aspire to moral standards that are so high that it is difficult for you to realize goals?*

  b. Inclusion: Also requires impairment in interpersonal functioning as manifested by at least <u>one</u> of the following difficulties.

    i. Empathy: *Do you struggle to understand and appreciate the ideas, feelings, or behaviors of other people?*

    ii. Intimacy: *In comparison to your work life, do you usually perceive relationships as secondary, or a lower priority? Does your need to be right or to not change your position frequently make it difficult to make and maintain relationships with other people?*

c. Inclusion: Also requires pathological personality traits from <u>both</u> of the following domains.

i. Compulsivity, characterized by the following:

- Rigid perfectionism: *Do you usually insist on things in your life being flawless, perfect, or without errors or fault? Do you frequently sacrifice finishing an activity or project on time in order to make sure every detail is correct? Do you usually believe there is only one right way to do things? Do you have a difficult time altering your ideas or viewpoint, even when you become aware of a compelling alternative? Are you preoccupied with details, organization, and order?*

ii. Negative affectivity, characterized by the following:

- Perseveration: *Do you frequently continue working on a task long after doing so is no longer effective? Do you frequently continue the same behaviors even after they have repeatedly resulted in failure?*

d. Exclusions

i. If the impairments in personality functioning and the expression of personality traits are unstable over time and inconsistent across situations, do not make the diagnosis.

ii. If the impairments in personality functioning and the personality trait expressions are normative for a person's developmental stage or sociocultural environment, do not make the diagnosis.

iii. If the impairments in personality functioning and the personality trait expressions are solely associated with the direct physiological effects of another medical condition or a substance, do not make the diagnosis.

e. Modifiers

i. Descriptive features

- More pervasive negative affectivity
- More pervasive detachment
- More pervasive antagonism

- More pervasive disinhibition
- More pervasive psychoticism
- Level of personality functioning (0–4) (see Level of Personality Functioning Scale in this chapter)

   f. Alternative: If a person exhibits significant impairment in self and interpersonal functioning but does not meet criteria for a specific personality disorder, consider personality disorder—trait specified (full proposed criteria are in DSM-5, pp. 770). The diagnosis allows you to specify the domains in which pathological personality domains—negative affectivity, detachment, antagonism, disinhibition, and psychoticism—are present and to diagnose the disorder. If you desire, you can use the specific trait facets within each domain to particularize the diagnosis. (You can see a list of these facets in the Personality Trait Rating Form on p. 222 of this chapter.)

3. Avoidant Personality Disorder

   a. Inclusion: Requires impairments in self-functioning as manifested by at least <u>one</u> of the following difficulties.

      i. Identity: *Do you have such low self-esteem that you usually perceive yourself as socially inept, unappealing, or inferior to other people? Do you frequently experience painful feelings of humiliation or inadequacy when you consider yourself?*

      ii. Self-direction: *Do you set such unrealistic standards for your behavior that it makes you reluctant to pursue your goals, take personal risks, or engage in new activities that would require you to interact with other people?*

   b. Inclusion: Also requires impairment in interpersonal functioning as manifested by at least <u>one</u> of the following difficulties.

      i. Empathy: *Do you frequently find that your thoughts are dominated by the possibility that other people will criticize or reject you?*

      ii. Intimacy: *Are you usually reluctant to become involved with other people unless you can be certain they will like you? Do you find it hard to make and maintain relationships because you fear being ridiculed or shamed?*

c. Inclusion: Also requires pathological personality traits from <u>all</u> of the following domains.

   i. Detachment, characterized by at least <u>one</u> of the following:

- Withdrawal: *In social situations, are you usually reserved, often to the point of not communicating unless it is necessary? Do you avoid social activity? Do you rarely begin or initiate social contact?*
- Intimacy avoidance: *Do you usually avoid close or romantic relationships, interpersonal attachments, and intimate sexual relationships?*
- Anhedonia: *Do you find it hard to be engaged in, or have energy for, life experiences? Do you find it difficult to feel pleasure?*

   ii. Negative affectivity, characterized by the following:

- Anxiousness: *Do you frequently experience intense feelings of nervousness, tension, or panic, often in reaction to social situations? Do you often worry about the negative effects of unpleasant experiences from your past and how they might affect your future? When you confront a situation that is uncertain or unsettled, do you often feel fearful, apprehensive, or threatened?*

d. Exclusions

   i. If the impairments in personality functioning and the expression of personality traits are unstable over time and inconsistent across situations, do not make the diagnosis.

   ii. If the impairments in personality functioning and the personality trait expressions are normative for a person's developmental stage or sociocultural environment, do not make the diagnosis.

   iii. If the impairments in personality functioning and the personality trait expressions are solely associated with the direct physiological effects of another medical condition or a substance, do not make the diagnosis.

e. Modifiers

   i. Descriptive features

- More pervasive negative affectivity
- More pervasive detachment

- More pervasive antagonism
- More pervasive disinhibition
- More pervasive psychoticism
- Level of personality functioning (0–4) (see Level of Personality Functioning Scale in this chapter)

f. Alternative: If a person exhibits significant impairment in self-functioning and interpersonal functioning, but does not meet criteria for a specific personality disorder, consider personality disorder—trait specified (full criteria are in DSM-5, p. 770). The diagnosis allows you to specify the domains in which pathological personality domains—negative affectivity, detachment, antagonism, disinhibition, and psychoticism—are present and to diagnose the disorder. If you desire, you can use the specific trait facets within each domain to particularize the diagnosis. (You can see a list of these facets in the Personality Trait Rating Form on p. 222 of this chapter.)

4. Schizotypal Personality Disorder

a. Inclusion: Requires impairments in self-functioning as manifested by at least <u>one</u> of the following difficulties.

i. Identity: *Do you often find yourself confused about the boundaries between yourself and other people? Do other people ever tell you that you seem indifferent or aloof?*

ii. Self-direction: *Do you frequently find it difficult to make realistic or coherent goals?*

b. Inclusion: Also requires impairment in interpersonal functioning as manifested by at least <u>one</u> of the following difficulties.

i. Empathy: *Do you often find it difficult to understand how your behaviors affect other people? Do you often find that you misunderstand other people's behaviors and motivations?*

ii. Intimacy: *Are you so anxious or distrustful of other people that you struggle to make close friendships or other relationships?*

c. Inclusion: Also requires pathological personality traits from at least <u>one</u> of the following domains.

i. Psychoticism, characterized by at least <u>one</u> of the following:

- Eccentricity: *Do other people often respond to you as if your behavior or appearance was odd or bizarre? Do other people often tell you that the things you say are inappropriate or unusual?*
- Cognitive and perceptual dysregulation: Odd or unusual thought processes; vague, circumstantial, metaphorical, overelaborate, or stereotyped thought or speech; odd sensations in various modalities. *Do other people often have trouble following your thought process? Do other people often struggle to understand your speech? Do you often experience odd sensations, like the feeling that something unnatural is on your skin or inside your body, or that you see or hear things other people cannot?*
- Unusual beliefs and experiences: *Do you sometimes have the sense that another person, whom other people cannot see, is present and speaking with you? Are you very superstitious? Are you preoccupied with paranormal or magical phenomena?*

ii. Detachment, characterized by at least <u>one</u> of the following:

- Restricted affectivity: *Do you notice that your emotional experiences and expressions stay within a narrow range and do not change much over time? Have other people told you that you do not respond to emotionally provocative situations as they expect? Have other people ever told you that you seem emotionally cold or indifferent?*
- Withdrawal: *Do you usually prefer to be alone? In social situations, are you usually reserved, often to the point of not communicating unless it is necessary? Do you avoid social activity? Do you rarely begin or initiate social contact?*

iii. Negative affectivity, characterized by the following:

- Suspiciousness: *Do you frequently doubt that other people will be faithful, loyal, and supportive of you? Do you often suspect that other people have negative or harmful intentions toward you? Do you often feel like other people are persecuting you?*

d. Exclusions

    i. If the impairments in personality functioning and the expression of personality traits are unstable over time and inconsistent across situations, do not make the diagnosis.

    ii. If the impairments in personality functioning and the personality trait expressions are normative for a person's developmental stage or sociocultural environment, do not make the diagnosis.

    iii. If the impairments in personality functioning and the personality trait expressions are solely associated with the direct physiological effects of another medical condition or a substance, do not make the diagnosis.

e. Modifiers

    i. Descriptive features

- More pervasive negative affectivity
- More pervasive detachment
- More pervasive antagonism
- More pervasive disinhibition
- More pervasive psychoticism
- Level of personality functioning (0–4) (see Level of Personality Functioning Scale in this chapter)

f. Alternative: If a person exhibits significant impairment in self and interpersonal functioning but does not meet criteria for a specific personality disorder, consider personality disorder—trait specified (full proposed criteria are in DSM-5, p. 770). The diagnosis allows you to specify the domains in which pathological personality domains—negative affectivity, detachment, antagonism, disinhibition, and psychoticism—are present and to diagnose the disorder. If you desire, you can use the specific trait facets within each domain to particularize the diagnosis. (You can see a list of these facets in the Personality Trait Rating Form on p. 222 of this chapter.)

5. Antisocial (Dissocial) Personality Disorder

a. Inclusion: Requires impairments in self-functioning as manifested by at least <u>one</u> of the following difficulties.

    i. Identity: *When you think about what makes you feel proud of yourself, do you find that it is usually personal* gain, pleasure, or the attainment and exercise of power? When you are making choices, do you usually think of how they will affect you more than how they will affect other people?

   ii. Self-direction: *When you set short- and long-term goals, is your chief motivation to gratify your own needs and desires? How important is it to you that your goals follow commonly accepted rules and guidelines for what is ethical and legal?*

  b. Inclusion: Also requires impairment in interpersonal functioning as manifested by at least <u>one</u> of the following difficulties.

   i. Empathy: *How concerned are you about the feelings, needs, or suffering of other people? If you have ever hurt or mistreated someone else, did you feel remorse or regret after doing so?*

   ii. Intimacy: *Do you find that you are incapable of being in relationships with other people in which you are emotionally close and engaged? Have you often coerced, deceived, exploited, or intimidated other people in an effort to control them?*

  c. Inclusion: Also requires pathological personality traits from <u>all</u> of the following domains.

   i. Antagonism, characterized by at least <u>one</u> of the following:

- Manipulativeness: *Do you frequently charm or seduce other people to achieve something you desire? Do you frequently deceive other people in order to influence or control them?*
- Deceitfulness: *Do you often misrepresent yourself by claiming accomplishments or qualities that are not your own? Do you often embellish stories and make up events?*
- Callousness: *When you hear about other people's feelings or problems, do you usually feel disinterested or unsympathetic? When you learn that your own actions have harmed someone else, do you feel guilty afterward? Do you find it pleasurable to inflict pain and suffering on another person?*
- Hostility: *Are you frequently or even always angry? When someone slights or insults you, does it often make you irritable or even aggressive? Are you often rude, nasty, or vengeful?*

ii. Disinhibition, characterized by at least <u>one</u> of the following:

- Irresponsibility: *When you enter into agreements or make promises, do you often disrespect and fail to follow through on your commitments? When you have familial, financial, and other obligations, do you often disregard and fail to honor them?*
- Impulsivity: *Do you often struggle to formulate and follow a plan? Do you often act on the spur of the moment, without a plan or consideration of the consequences?*
- Risk taking: *Do you often engage in dangerous, risky, and potentially self-damaging activities with little thought to the consequences? Are you easily bored, and do you often start activities without thinking as a way to counter your boredom?*

d. Exclusions

i. If the impairments in personality functioning and the expression of personality traits are unstable over time and inconsistent across situations, do not make the diagnosis.

ii. If the impairments in personality functioning and the personality trait expressions are normative for a person's developmental stage or sociocultural environment, do not make the diagnosis.

iii. If the impairments in personality functioning and the personality trait expressions are solely associated with the direct physiological effects of another medical condition or a substance, do not make the diagnosis.

e. Modifiers

i. Descriptive features

- More pervasive negative affectivity
- More pervasive detachment
- More pervasive antagonism
- More pervasive disinhibition
- More pervasive psychoticism
- Level of personality functioning (0–4) (see Level of Personality Functioning Scale in this chapter)

ii. Specifiers

- With psychopathic features specifier: Use when a person exhibits a lack of anxiety or fear and a bold, efficacious interpersonal style. Psychopathy comparatively emphasizes affective and interpersonal characteristics over the behavioral components.

f. Alternative: If a person exhibits significant impairment in self-functioning and interpersonal functioning but does not meet criteria for a specific personality disorder, consider personality disorder—trait specified (full proposed criteria are in DSM-5, p. 770). The diagnosis allows you to specify the domains in which pathological personality domains—negative affectivity, detachment, antagonism, disinhibition, and psychoticism—are present and to diagnose the disorder. If you desire, you can use the specific trait facets within each domain to particularize the diagnosis. (You can see a list of these facets in the Personality Trait Rating Form on p. 222 of this chapter.)

6. Narcissistic Personality Disorder

a. Inclusion: Requires impairments in self-functioning as manifested by at least <u>one</u> of the following difficulties.

i. Identity: *Do you define yourself mostly in relationship to other people? Does the pride you take in yourself depend on how other people perceive and respond to you? Do you find that your emotions fluctuate in response to your estimation of the quality of your life?*

ii. Self-direction: *Do you find it hard to understand what motivates you to make decisions and set goals? Do you usually set goals for yourself based on how other people will perceive your goals? Do you set standards for yourself really high to reflect how exceptional you are? Alternatively, do you set standards for yourself really low to reflect that you are entitled to whatever you achieve?*

b. Inclusion: Also requires impairment in interpersonal functioning as manifested by at least <u>one</u> of the following difficulties.

i. Empathy: *Are you very attuned to the reactions other people have to you? Do you frequently think about how you affect other people? Do you find it hard to recognize or identify with the feelings and needs of other people?*

    ii. Intimacy: *In your relationships with other people, do you find that you are interested in other people and their experiences in terms of what they mean to you and your life? Do most of your relationships stay casual or on the surface? Do you value relationships with other people as a way to maintain your self-esteem?*

c. Inclusion: Also requires pathological personality traits from this domain.

    i. Antagonism, characterized by <u>both</u> of the following:

- Grandiosity: *Do you deserve or have a right to particular treatments because of your excellent personal qualities? Do you believe that you are better or superior to other people? Do you often act in a way that makes other people inferior to you?*
- Attention seeking: *Do you really like being the center of attention? Do you find that you often seek and attract the attention or admiration of other people?*

d. Exclusions

    i. If the impairments in personality functioning and the expression of personality traits are unstable over time and inconsistent across situations, do not make the diagnosis.

    ii. If the impairments in personality functioning and the personality trait expressions are normative for a person's developmental stage or sociocultural environment, do not make the diagnosis.

    iii. If the impairments in personality functioning and the personality trait expressions are solely associated with the direct physiological effects of another medical condition or a substance, do not make the diagnosis.

e. Modifiers

    i. Descriptive features

- More pervasive negative affectivity
- More pervasive detachment
- More pervasive antagonism
- More pervasive disinhibition
- More pervasive psychoticism

- Level of personality functioning (0–4)
  (see Level of Personality Functioning Scale
  in this chapter)

f. Alternative: If a person exhibits significant impairment in self-functioning and interpersonal functioning but does not meet criteria for a specific personality disorder, consider personality disorder—trait specified (full criteria are in DSM-5, p. 770). The diagnosis allows you to specify the domains in which pathological personality domains—negative affectivity, detachment, antagonism, disinhibition, and psychoticism—are present and to diagnose the disorder. If you desire, you can use the specific trait facets within each domain to particularize the diagnosis. (You can see a list of these facets in the Personality Trait Rating Form on p. 222 of this chapter.)

Chapter 13

Alternative Diagnostic Systems and Rating Scales

DSM-5 provides a common language for characterizing the mental distress a person experiences. However, it is not the only common language. In various communities, alternative languages may be widely spoken. Although I cannot fully consider these languages in this book, I discuss a few notable alternatives, along with diagnosis-specific rating scales.

Alternative Diagnostic Systems

International Classification of Diseases

The World Health Organization maintains its own diagnostic system, the International Classification of Diseases, commonly known by its abbreviation, ICD. The current, tenth edition, or ICD-10, includes mental disorders among a catalog of all medical diseases. The eleventh edition is expected in 2014, and dialogue is occurring to synchronize ICD-11 and DSM-5 (Andrews et al. 2009). Although most clinicians outside the United States use ICD-10 to diagnose mental disorders, ICD-10 is less detailed than DSM-5 and was primarily designed to help epidemiologists track the incidence and prevalence of disease. Despite their different designs, DSM and ICD-10 assign the same codes to psychiatric diagnoses, and these shared codes are widely used by insurers. You can find information about ICD-10 and a list of diagnostic codes at www.who.int/classifications/icd/en/. The fifth chapter, "Mental and Behavioural Disorders," includes most of the diagnoses relevant for the diagnostic interview.

Psychodynamic Diagnostic Manual

ICD-10 is focused on public health, whereas the *Psychodynamic Diagnostic Manual* (PDM; Alliance of Psychoanalytic Organizations 2006) focuses on the psychological health and distress of a particular person. Several psychoanalytical groups joined together to create PDM as a complement to the descriptive systems of DSM-5 and ICD-10. Like DSM-5, PDM includes dimensions that cut across diagnostic categories, along with a thorough account of personality patterns and disorders. PDM uses the DSM diagnostic categories but includes accounts of the internal experience of a person presenting for treatment. You can read more about PDM at www.pdm1.org.

McHugh's Clusters

Over the past several decades, the psychiatrist Paul McHugh has expressed frustration at how DSM separated the symptoms from the cause of a mental illness. McHugh argues that by ignoring the putative cause of a disorder, DSM discourages attempts to understand a disorder (McHugh and Slaveny 2012). As an alternative, McHugh proposes grouping mental illnesses into four "clusters" based on the cause of a person's distress. McHugh correlates each cluster with metaphors for treatment. In his first cluster, McHugh includes structural brain diseases that directly disturb psychological functioning; these can be described roughly as what a person *has*. This cluster includes disorders such as Alzheimer's disease, delirium, and schizophrenia. For persons with these illnesses, practitioners seek a cure. In his second cluster, McHugh (2005) includes psychological troubles that result from the way someone's mind matured, as in most personality disorders, or roughly who a person *is*. For persons with these illnesses, practitioners act as guides. In the third cluster, he includes disturbances that result from biologically reinforced behaviors such as substance abuse and anorexia nervosa, or what a person *does*. For persons with these illnesses, practitioners interrupt the behavior. In the fourth cluster, he includes distress due to events that endanger a person's identity, such as bereavement and posttraumatic stress disorder, or what a person *encounters*. For persons with these illnesses, the practitioner helps a person rescript his life story. Although McHugh's diagnostic system has not been widely adopted, his observations have been influential and are accessible reading for anyone interested in the meaning of psychiatric diagnosis and classification (McHugh and Slaveny 1998).

Research Domain Criteria

In 2010, the National Institute of Mental Health announced its intention to produce its own diagnostic system, the Research Domain Criteria (RDoC), which will similarly unite symptoms with their cause. RDoC has not yet been written, but it is intended to be a neuroscience-informed nosology in which behaviors are mapped onto specific, interrelated circuits of the brain. Instead of characterizing a mental disorder by its symptoms, RDoC will characterize a disorder by the affected neural circuits. For example, anxious worry might be described as a disorder of a particular cortical-striatal-thalamic-cortical circuit. RDoC assumes that neural circuits can be identified by the tools of clinical neuroscience, but acknowledges that some of these tools and techniques have not yet been produced. Therefore, although RDoC remains an aspiration rather than a clinical reality, it is considered the future of psychiatric diagnosis. In a way, DSM-5 takes an important step in the direction of RDoC because it includes dimensions, which are analogous to what the RDoC calls behavioral "domains," such as impulsivity and negative emotionality, which cut across contemporary diagnostic categories, and renews consideration of the etiology of mental distress (Insel and Quirion 2005; Insel et al. 2010). You can follow the progress of the development of RDoC at this URL: www.nimh.nih.gov/research-funding/rdoc/index.shtml.

Culture-Specific Diagnostic Systems

In addition, there are several culture-specific psychiatric diagnostic systems that are used in particular communities, including Latin America (Berganza et al. 2002), Cuba (Otero-Ojeda 2002), China (Chen 2002), and Japan (Nakane and Nakane 2002).

Rating Scales

Clinicians and researchers have created many rating scales to quantify degrees of health, illness, and impairment. Because the authors of many of these rating scales have copyrighted the scales, not all of them are freely available. You can find a good, albeit incomplete, list of rating scales at this URL: www.neurotransmitter.net/ratingscales.html.

References

Alarcón RD, Frank JB: The Psychotherapy of Hope: The Legacy of Persuasion and Healing. Baltimore, MD, Johns Hopkins University Press, 2011

Alliance of Psychoanalytic Organizations: Psychodynamic Diagnostic Manual. Silver Spring, MD, Alliance of Psychoanalytic Organizations, 2006

American Psychiatric Association: Diagnostic and Statistical Manual of Mental Disorders, 3rd Edition. Washington, DC, American Psychiatric Association, 1980

American Psychiatric Association: Diagnostic and Statistical Manual of Mental Disorders, 4th Edition, Text Revision. Washington, DC, American Psychiatric Association, 2000

American Psychiatric Association: The Principles of Medical Ethics: With Annotations Especially Applicable to Psychiatry. Washington, DC, American Psychiatric Association, 2010

American Psychiatric Association: Diagnostic and Statistical Manual of Mental Disorders, 5th Edition. Washington, DC, American Psychiatric Association, 2013

Andrews G, Goldberg DP, Krueger RF, et al: Exploring the feasibility of a meta-structure for DSM-5 and ICD-11: could it improve utility and validity? Psychol Med 39:1993–2000, 2009

Aragona M: The concept of mental disorder and the DSM-5. Dialogues in Philosophy, Mental and Neuro Sciences 2:1–14, 2009

Bäärnhielm S, Rosso MS: The cultural formulation: a model to combine nosology and patients' life context in psychiatric diagnostic practice. Transcult Psychiatry 46:406–428, 2009

Barnhill JW (ed): DSM-5 Clinical Cases. Washington, DC, American Psychiatric Publishing, 2014

Bentall RP: A proposal to classify happiness as a psychiatric disorder. J Med Ethics 18:94–98, 1992

Berganza CE, Mezzich JE, Jorge MR: Latin American Guide for Psychiatric Diagnosis (GLDP). Psychopathology 35:185–190, 2002

Black DW, Grant JE: DSM-5 Guidebook: The Essential Companion to the Diagnostic and Statistical Manual of Mental Disorders, 5th Edition. Washington, DC, American Psychiatric Publishing, 2014

Carlat DJ: The Psychiatric Interview, 2nd Edition. Philadelphia, PA, Lippincott, Williams & Wilkins, 2005

Cassell EJ: The Nature of Suffering and the Goals of Medicine. New York, Oxford University Press, 1991

Chen YF: Chinese Classification of Mental Disorders (CCMD-3). Psychopathology 35:171–175, 2002

Davies O: A Theology of Compassion: Metaphysics of Difference and the Renewal of Tradition. Grand Rapids, MI, William B Eerdmans, 2001

Digman JM: Personality structure: emergence of the five-factor model. Annu Rev Psychol 41:417–440, 1990

Emanuel EJ, Emanuel LL: Four models of the physician-patient relationship. JAMA 267:2221–2226, 1992

Estroff SE, Henderson GE: Social and cultural contributions to health, difference, and inequality, in The Social Medicine Reader, 2nd Edition, Vol 2. Durham, NC, Duke University Press, 2005, pp 4–26

Fairburn CG, Bohn K: Eating disorder NOS (EDNOS): an example of the troublesome "not otherwise specified" (NOS) category in DSM-IV. Behav Res Ther 43:691–701, 2005

Feinstein AR: Clinical Judgment. Baltimore, MD, Williams & Wilkins, 1967

First MB: DSM-5 Handbook of Differential Diagnosis. Washington, DC, American Psychiatric Publishing, 2014

Frank JD, Frank JB: Persuasion and Healing: A Comparative Study of Psychotherapy, 3rd Edition. Baltimore, MD, Johns Hopkins University Press, 1991

Goldman HH, Skodol AE, Lave TR: Revising Axis V for DSM-IV: a review of measures of social functioning. Am J Psychiatry 149:1148–1156, 1992

Grob GN: Origins of DSM-I: a study in appearance and reality. Am J Psychiatry 148:421–431, 1991

Houts AC: Fifty years of psychiatric nomenclature: reflections on the 1943 War Department Technical Bulletin, Medical 203. J Clin Psychol 56:935–967, 2000

Hunter KM: How Doctors Think: Clinical Judgment and the Practice of Medicine. New York, Oxford University Press, 2005

Insel T, Quirion R: Psychiatry as a clinical neuroscience discipline. JAMA 294:2221–2224, 2005

Insel T, Cuthbert B, Garvey M, et al: Research Domain Criteria (RDoC): toward a new classification framework for research on mental disorders. Am J Psychiatry 167:748–751, 2010

Johnson RL, Sadosty AT, Weaver AL, et al: To sit or not to sit? Ann Emerg Med 51:188–193, 2008

Kendell R, Jablensky A: Distinguishing between the validity and utility of psychiatric diagnoses. Am J Psychiatry 160:4–12, 2003

Kendler KS: The dappled nature of causes of psychiatric illness: replacing the organic-functional/hardware-software dichotomy with empirically based pluralism. Mol Psychiatry 17:377–388, 2012

Kernberg OF: Severe Personality Disorders. New Haven, CT, Yale University Press, 1984

King LS: Medical Thinking: A Historical Preface. Princeton, NJ, Princeton University Press, 1982

Kinghorn WA: Whose disorder? A constructive MacIntyrean critique of psychiatric nosology. J Med Philos 36:187–205, 2011

Kleinman A, Eisenberg L, Good B: Culture, illness, and care: critical lessons from anthropologic and cross-cultural research. Ann Intern Med 88:251–258, 1978

Kupfer DJ, Regier DA: Why all of medicine should care about DSM-5. JAMA 303:1974–1975, 2010

Kupfer DJ, Regier DA: Neuroscience, clinical evidence, and the future of psychiatric classification in DSM-5. Am J Psychiatry 168:672–674, 2011

Lewis-Fernández R, Hinton DE, Laria AJ: Culture and the anxiety disorders: recommendations for DSM-5. Depress Anxiety 27:212–229, 2010

Little M: Talking cure and curing talk. J R Soc Med 98:210–212, 2005

Lizardi D, Oquendo MA, Graver R: Clinical pitfalls in the diagnosis of ataque de nervios: a case study. Transcult Psychiatry 46:463–486, 2009

MacKinnon RA, Michels R, Buckley PJ: The Psychiatric Interview in Clinical Practice, 2nd Edition. Washington, DC, American Psychiatric Publishing, 2006

Martínez LC: DSM-IV-TR cultural formulation of psychiatric cases: two proposals for clinicians. Transcult Psychiatry 46:506–523, 2009

McHugh PR: Striving for coherence: psychiatry's efforts over classification. JAMA 293:2526–2528, 2005

McHugh P: Review of "The Loss of Sadness: How Psychiatry Transformed Normal Sorrow Into Depressive Disorder." N Engl J Med 357:947–948, 2007

McHugh P, Slaveny PR: The Perspectives of Psychiatry, 2nd Edition. Baltimore, MD, Johns Hopkins University Press, 1998

McHugh P, Slaveny PR: Mental illness—comprehensive evaluation or checklist? N Engl J Med 366:1853–1855, 2012

Morrison J, Muñoz RA: Boarding Time: The Psychiatry Candidate's New Guide to Part II of the ABPN Examination. Washington, DC, American Psychiatric Publishing, 2009

Mundt C, Backenstrass M: Psychotherapy and classification: psychological, psychodynamic, and cognitive aspects. Psychopathology 38:219–222, 2005

Nakane Y, Nakane H: Classification systems for psychiatric diseases currently used in Japan. Psychopathology 35:191–194, 2002

Oliver N (writer): Lars and the Real Girl. Los Angeles, CA, Lars Productions, 2007

Otero-Ojeda AA: Third Cuban Glossary of Psychiatry (GC-3): key features and contributions. Psychopathology 35:181–184, 2002

Parsons T: Illness and the role of the physician: a sociological perspective. Am J Orthopsychiatry 21:452–460, 1951

Phillips J, Frances A, Cerullo MA, et al: The six most essential questions in psychiatric diagnosis: a pluralogue part 1: conceptual and definitional issues in psychiatric diagnosis. Philos Ethics Humanit Med 7:3, 2012a

Phillips J, Frances A, Cerullo MA, et al: The six most essential questions in psychiatric diagnosis: a pluralogue part 2: issues of conservatism and pragmatism in psychiatric diagnosis. Philos Ethics Humanit Med 7:8, 2012b

Phillips J, Frances A, Cerullo MA, et al: The six most essential questions in psychiatric diagnosis: a pluralogue part 3: issues of utility and alternative approaches in psychiatric diagnosis. Philos Ethics Humanit Med 7:9, 2012c

Pierre J: The borders of mental disorders in psychiatry and the DSM: past, present, and future. J Psychiatr Pract 16:375–386, 2010

Radden J, Sadler JZ: The Virtuous Psychiatrist: Character Ethics in Psychiatric Practice. New York, Oxford University Press, 2010

Regier DA: Dimensional approaches to psychiatric classification: refining the research agenda for DSM-5: an introduction. Int J Methods Psychiatr Res 16(suppl 1):1–5, 2007

Regier DA, Narrow WE, Kuhl EA, et al: The conceptual development of DSM-5. Am J Psychiatry 166:645–650, 2009

Roberts LW, Louie AK: Study Guide to DSM-5. Washington, DC, American Psychiatric Publishing, 2014

Robertson K: Active listening: more than just paying attention. Aust Fam Physician 34:1053–1055, 2005

Rondeau E, Klein LS, Masse A, et al: Is pervasive developmental disorder not otherwise specified less stable than autistic disorder? A meta-analysis. J Autism Dev Disord 41:1267–1276, 2011

Rosenhan DL: On being sane in insane places. Science 179:250–258, 1973

Rüsch N, Angermeyer MC, Corrigan PW: Mental illness stigma: concepts, consequences, and initiatives to reduce stigmas. Eur Psychiatry 20:529–539, 2005

Shahrokh NC, Hales RE, Phillips KA, et al: The Language of Mental Health: A Glossary of Psychiatric Terms. Washington, DC, American Psychiatric Publishing, 2011

Shea SC: Psychiatric Interviewing: The Art of Understanding, 2nd Edition. Philadelphia, PA, WB Saunders, 1998

Shweder RA: Why Do Men Barbecue? Recipes for Cultural Psychology. Cambridge, MA, Harvard University Press, 2003

Spitzer RL: Values and assumptions in the development of DSM-III and DSM-III-R: an insider's perspective and a belated response to Sadler, Hulgus, and Agich's "On values in recent American psychiatric classification." J Nerv Ment Dis 189:351–359, 2001

Stein DJ, Phillips KA, Bolton D, et al: What is a mental/psychiatric disorder? From DSM-IV to DSM-5. Psychol Med 40:1759–1765, 2010

Sullivan HS: The Collected Works of Harry Stack Sullivan, Vol 1: The Psychiatric Interview. Edited by Perry HS, Gawel ML. New York, WW Norton, 1954

Summers RF, Barber JP: Therapeutic alliance as a measurable psychotherapy skill. Acad Psychiatry 27:160–165, 2003

Wallace ER: Psychiatry and its nosology: a historico-philosophical overview, in Philosophical Perspective on Psychiatric Diagnostic Classification. Edited by Sadler JZ, Wiggins OP, Schwartz MA. Baltimore, MD, Johns Hopkins University Press, 1994, pp 16–88

Weiden PJ: Understanding and addressing adherence issues in schizophrenia: from theory to practice. J Clin Psychiatry 68(suppl 14):14–19, 2007

Wiggins OP, Schwartz MA: The limits of psychiatric knowledge and the problem of classification, in Philosophical Perspective on Psychiatric Diagnostic Classification. Edited by Sadler JZ, Wiggins OP, Schwartz MA. Baltimore, MD, Johns Hopkins University Press, 1994, pp 89–103

Wilson M: DSM-III and the transformation of American psychiatry: a history. Am J Psychiatry 150:399–410, 1993

World Health Organization: International Statistical Classification of Diseases and Related Health Problems, 10th Revision. Geneva, World Health Organization, 1992

World Health Organization: Measuring Health and Disability: Manual for WHO Disability Assessment Schedule (WHODAS 2.0). Edited by Üstün TB, Kostanjsek N, Chatterji S, et al. Geneva, World Health Organization, 2010

Yager J: Specific components of bedside manner in the general hospital psychiatric consultation: 12 concrete suggestions. Psychosomatics 30:209–212, 1989

Zimmerman M: Interview Guide for Evaluating DSM-IV Psychiatric Disorders and the Mental Status Examination. East Greenwich, RI, Psych Products Press, 1994

Index

Page numbers printed in **boldface** *type refer to tables or figures.*

Anger *(continued)*
    depressive disorders in
        children and, 80
    tobacco withdrawal and, 154
Anhedonia, and personality
    disorders, **224,** 233
Anorexia nervosa, 35, 101–103
Antagonism, and personality
    disorders, 49, **224,** 227,
    229, 237, 240
Antisocial personality disorder,
    169, 227, 236–239
Anxiety. *See also* Anxiety
    disorders
    avoidant personality
        disorder and, 233
    borderline personality
        disorder and, 228
    cannabis withdrawal and,
        136
    DSM-IV-TR and, 33
    illness anxiety disorder and,
        100
    Personality Trait Rating
        Form and, **223**
    sedative, hypnotic, or
        anxiolytic withdrawal
        and, 148
    somatic symptom disorder
        and, 98
    specific phobia and, 82
    30-minute diagnostic
        interview and questions
        on, 24
    tobacco withdrawal and, 154
Anxiety disorders, 82–86, **196.**
    See also Anxiety; Illness
    anxiety disorder
Aphonia, 204
Appearance
    histrionic personality
        disorder and, 171
    mental status examination
        and, 203

Appetite. *See also* Eating and
    feeding
    cannabis intoxication and,
        136
    cannabis withdrawal and,
        137
    stimulant withdrawal and,
        152
    tobacco withdrawal and,
        154
Arrogance, and narcissistic
    personality disorder,
    172
Art, formation of therapeutic
    alliance as, 15
Ataque de nervios, 38
Atheoretic principle, 5
Attention-deficit/hyperactivity
    disorder, 65–67, **194**
Attention seeking
    narcissistic personality
        disorder and, 48–49,
        227, 240
    Personality Trait Rating
        Form and, **224**
Autism spectrum disorder,
    62–65, **194**
Avoidance, and specific
    phobia, 82. *See also*
    Withdrawal
Avoidant personality disorder,
    172–173, 227, 232–233
Avoidant/restrictive food
    intake disorder, 103–104

Behavior. *See also* Aggression;
    Disinhibition; Eccentricity;
    Repetitive behaviors; Risk
    taking; Stereotypic
    behavior
    clinical significance versus
        "normality" of, 201–202
    mental status examination
        and, 203

Encopresis, 105–106
Enteral feeding, and avoidant/
    restrictive food intake
    disorder, 103
Entitlement, and narcissistic
    personality disorder, 172
Enuresis, 105
Environmental problems,
    codes for in ICD-9 and
    ICD-10, 180–189
Envy, and narcissistic
    personality disorder, 172
Episode, definition of, 42
Erectile disorder, 115–116
Euphoria, and inhalant
    intoxication, 142
Exclusion criteria. *See*
    Symptoms; *specific
    disorders*
Excoriation, 89
Exhibitionistic disorder, 176,
    177
Exploitation, and narcissistic
    personality disorder, 172

Factitious disorder, 99, 199
Family history, and 30-minute
    diagnostic interview, 26
Fantasies, and narcissistic
    personality disorder, 171
Fatigue
    caffeine withdrawal and,
        134
    depressive disorders and, 77
    generalized anxiety disorder
        and, 86
    stimulant withdrawal and,
        152
Fear
    panic disorder and, 84
    reactive attachment disorder
        and, 93
    specific phobia and, 82
    thought content and, 204

Feeding and eating disorders,
    and diagnostic interview,
    101–104. *See also* Anorexia
    nervosa; Eating and
    feeding
Female orgasmic disorder,
    116–117
Female sexual interest/arousal
    disorder, 117–119
Fetishistic disorder, 177, 178
Fever, and opioid withdrawal,
    145
Finances and financial
    situations. *See also*
    Psychosocial problems
    gambling disorder and, 157
    obsessive-compulsive
        personality disorder
        and, 174
Five-Factor Model, and
    personality disorders, 49
Flashbacks, and posttraumatic
    stress disorder, 90
Forgetfulness, and attention-
    deficit/hyperactivity
    disorder, 65. *See also*
    Memory
Frank, Jerome and Julia, 13–14,
    15
Frontotemporal lobar
    degeneration, 161
Frotteuristic disorder, 176

Gambling disorder, 157–158
Gastrointestinal disturbance,
    and caffeine intoxication,
    133
Gender, and use of terms,
    vii–viii
Gender dysphoria, and
    diagnostic interview,
    121–123
Generalized anxiety disorder,
    85–86, **196**

psychiatric diagnoses as threat to, 7

Illness, and concept of disorder, 6–8

Illness anxiety disorder, 100

Illusion, and thought content, 205

Impairment. *See also* Mental distress
body-focused repetitive behaviors and, 89
definition of mental disorder and, 9
differential diagnosis and, 202
Level of Personality Functioning Scale and, 216, **217–221**
narcissistic personality disorder and, 49, 50

Impulsivity
antisocial personality disorder and, 169, 238
attention-deficit/hyperactivity disorder and, 66, 67
borderline personality disorder and, 170, 229
Personality Trait Rating Form and, **225**

Inadequacy, and avoidant personality disorder, 172

Inattention, and attention-deficit/hyperactivity disorder, 65, 66. *See also* Distraction and distractibility

Inclusion criteria. *See* Symptoms; *specific disorders*

Incoordination
inhalant intoxication and, 141

phencyclidine or other hallucinogen intoxication and, 139

Inhalant intoxication, 141–142

Inhalant use disorder, 140–141

Insight, and obsessive-compulsive disorder, 88

Insomnia. *See also* Insomnia disorder; Sleep and sleep disturbance
alcohol withdrawal and, 132
caffeine intoxication and, 133
opioid withdrawal and, 145
sedative, hypnotic, or anxiolytic withdrawal and, 148
stimulant withdrawal and, 152
tobacco withdrawal and, 154

Insomnia disorder, 107–109

Intellectual disability, 59–62

Intellectual resources, and mental status examination, 205

Intermittent explosive disorder, 124–125

Interpersonal relationships. *See also* Intimacy; Withdrawal
autism spectrum disorder and, 62
avoidant personality disorder and, 172
borderline personality disorder and, 170
dependent personality disorder and, 173
histrionic personality disorder and, 171
Level of Personality Functioning Scale and, **217–221**
narcissistic personality disorder and, 48, 49, 50

Medical conditions, and differential diagnosis, 200–201. *See* Alternative diagnosis; *specific disorders*

Medical history
codes for psychosocial and environmental problems in record of, 180–189
30-minute diagnostic interview and, 26

Medication(s). *See also* Alternative diagnosis; Substance use
conditions resulting from adverse effects of, **179**
neurocognitive disorders and, 162
30-minute diagnostic interview and treatment plan, 30

Medication-induced movement disorders, **179**

Memory, and posttraumatic stress disorder, 90, 91. *See also* Forgetfulness

Mental disorders. *See* Disorders; *specific disorders*

Mental distress, and concept of *disorder*, 8, 202. *See also* Impairment

Mental status examination (MSE), 27, 203–205. *See also* Mini-Mental State Examination

Mild neurocognitive disorder, 163–164, **198**

Mind, and body in concept of *disorder*, 8

Mini-Mental State Examination (MMSE), 27, 159, 160

Misdiagnosis, risk of, 4

Modifiers. *See* Severity; *specific disorders*

Mood. *See also* Dysphoric mood; Emotions; Irritability
mental status examination and, 204
30-minute diagnostic interview and questions on, 24

Movement disorders, and adverse effects of medication, **179**

Multiaxial system, 8, 50–52

Muscle aches, and opioid withdrawal, 145

Muscle tension, and generalized anxiety disorder, 85

Mutism, 204. *See also* Selective mutism

Narcissistic personality disorder, 46–50, 171–172, 227, 239–241

Narcolepsy, 110–111

Narrative, and organization of patient presentation, 29

National Institute of Mental Health, 245

Nausea
alcohol withdrawal and, 132
opioid withdrawal and, 144
panic disorder and, 84
sedative, hypnotic, or anxiolytic withdrawal and, 148
stimulant intoxication and, 151

Negative symptoms, of schizophrenia, 68

Neologisms, 204

Nervousness, and caffeine intoxication, 133

Neurocognitive disorders, 159–164, **198**

Persecution, and thought content, 205
Perseveration, and personality disorders, **223**, 231
Persistent depressive disorder, 79
Persistent motor or vocal tic disorder, 64
Person, use of term, vii–vii
Personality, questions on in 30-minute diagnostic interview, 26. *See also* Personality Trait Rating Form
Personality disorders. *See also* Level of Personality Functioning Scale; Personality Trait Rating Form
diagnostic interviews for, 165–175, 227–241
dimensional diagnosis of, 47–50, 215
reconceptualization of, 36
systems for diagnosis of in DSM-5, 47
Personality Trait Rating Form, 50, 222, **223–226**, 230, 232, 234, 236, 239, 241
Perspiration, and stimulant intoxication, 151
Persuasion and Healing: A Comparative Study of Psychotherapy (Frank and Frank 1991), 13–14, 15
Phencyclidine or other hallucinogen intoxication, 139–140
Phencyclidine or other hallucinogen use disorder, 137–139
Phobias, 204. *See also* Specific phobia
Physical abuse. *See* Psychosocial problems

Physiological reactions, and posttraumatic stress disorder, 90–91. *See also* Somatic symptoms
Pica, 103
Point of view, and definition of mental disorder, 8
Polysomnography, and sleep disorders, 110, 111
Posttraumatic stress disorder, 90–92, **197**
Premature ejaculation, 116
Premenstrual dysphoric disorder, 79
Preoccupation
dependent personality disorder and, 173
gambling disorder and, 157
illness anxiety disorder and, 100
narcissistic personality disorder and, 171
obsessive-compulsive personality disorder and, 174
paranoid personality disorder and, 166
Prion disease, 162
Prognosis, and 30-minute diagnostic interview, 29
PROMIS Emotional Distress-Anxiety scale, 34
Provisional tic disorder, 64
Psychiatric history, and 30-minute diagnostic interview, 23
Psychiatric Interview in Clinical Practice, The (MacKinnon et al. 2006), 12
Psychodynamic Diagnostic Manual (Alliance of Psychoanalytic Organizations 2006), 243–244

Specific phobia, 82–84
Specifiers. *See specific disorders*
Speech, and mental status
    examination, 204
Speech sound disorder, 61
Stepwise approach, to
    differential diagnosis,
    199–202
Stereotypic behavior
    autism spectrum disorder
        and, 63
    mental status examination
        and, 205
Stereotypic movement
    disorder, 64
Stimulant intoxication, 151
Stimulant use disorder,
    149–150
Stimulant withdrawal, 151–152
Stress. *See* Trauma- and
    stressor-related disorders
Submissiveness, and
    Personality Trait Rating
    Form, **223**
Substance dependence, 45
Substance-related and
    addictive disorders, and
    diagnostic interviews,
    129–158
Substance use. *See also*
    Alternative diagnosis;
    Medication(s); Substance-
    related and addictive
    disorders; Withdrawal
    bipolar disorder and, 74
    depressive disorders and, 79
    differential diagnosis and,
        200
    neurocognitive disorders
        and, 162
    schizophrenia and, 70
    30-minute diagnostic
        interview and questions
        on, 25–26

Subtypes
    of anorexia nervosa, 101
    of conduct disorder, 126
    of delirium, 160
    of erectile disorder, 115
    of female orgasmic disorder,
        117
    of female sexual interest/
        arousal disorder, 118
    of illness anxiety disorder,
        100
    of major neurocognitive
        disorder, 161–163
    of male hypoactive sexual
        desire disorder, 119
    of mild neurocognitive
        disorder, 164
    of narcolepsy, 111
    of paraphilic disorders, 177
    of posttraumatic stress
        disorder, 92
    of schizophrenia, 44
Suggestibility, and histrionic
    personality disorder, 171
Suicide and suicidal ideation
    borderline personality
        disorder and, 170
    depressive disorders and,
        77–78
Support, and dependent
    personality disorder, 173
Suspiciousness
    paranoid personality
        disorder and, 166
    Personality Trait Rating
        Form and, **223**
    schizotypal personality
        disorder and, 168, 235
Symptoms. *See also* Age at
    onset; Duration; Negative
    symptoms; Psychosis and
    psychotic symptoms;
    Somatic symptoms;
    specific disorders

phencyclidine or other
hallucinogen
intoxication and, 139
Voyeuristic disorder, 176, 177

Weight loss or gain
anorexia nervosa and, 101
avoidant/restrictive food
intake disorder and, 103
depressive disorders and, 77
Withdrawal. *See also* Alcohol
withdrawal; Caffeine
withdrawal; Interpersonal
relationships; Opioid
withdrawal; Other (or
unknown) substance
withdrawal; Stimulant
withdrawal
alcohol use disorder and,
130
avoidant personality
disorder and, 233
caffeine withdrawal and, 135
opioid use disorder and, 143

other (or unknown)
substance use disorder
and, 155
Personality Trait Rating
Form and, **224**
schizotypal personality
disorder and, 235
stimulant use disorder and,
150
tobacco use disorder and,
153
World Health Organization,
243
World Health Organization
Disability Assessment
Schedule 2.0 (WHODAS
2.0), 9, 52, 211
Worry, and panic disorder, 85

Yager, Joel, 19
Yawning, and opioid
withdrawal, 145

Z codes. *See* ICD-10